PRENTICE-HALL
FOUNDATIONS OF IMMUNOLOGY SERIES

EDITORS

Abraham G. Osler

*The Public Health Research Institute of the City of New York
and New York University School of Medicine*

Leon Weiss

The Johns Hopkins University School of Medicine

THE IMMUNOBIOLOGY OF TRANSPLANTATION
Rupert E. Billingham and Willys Silvers

THE CELLS AND TISSUES OF THE IMMUNE SYSTEM
Leon Weiss

COMPLEMENT: MECHANISMS AND FUNCTIONS
Abraham G. Osler

THE IMMUNE SYSTEM OF SECRETIONS
Thomas B. Tomasi, Jr.

COMPARATIVE IMMUNOLOGY
Edwin L. Cooper

THE IMMUNOBIOLOGY OF MAMMALIAN REPRODUCTION
Alan E. Beer and Rupert E. Billingham

RADIOIMMUNOASSAY OF BIOLOGICALLY ACTIVE COMPOUNDS
Charles W. Parker

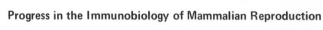

Progress in the Immunobiology of Mammalian Reproduction

The chronology of some major discoveries and concepts
in the immunology of mammalian reproduction

Immunologic control of sex ratio

Control of conception by "vaccination"

Egg transplantation in man

Natural "transplantation" of viable leukocytes from mother to
offspring via the milk in rats

Rh isoimmunization of Rh negative fetuses following natural
maternal to fetal transfer of erythrocytes

Experimental augmentation of maternal to fetal leukocyte
traffic resulting in sensitization, maternally induced tolerance,
and GVH disease

Recognition that heterospecific pregnancies induce regional
lymphadenopathy in many species

expression of H-LA antigens by human spermatozoa

Presence of fetal leukocytes in maternal circulation in women

Natural maternally induced GVH disease in rats

Allergy to human seminal plasma in a woman

Development of fatal GVH disease in infant following intrauterine
transfusion of adult donor blood

Selective effect associated with histocompatibility locus in
the rat

Recognition of natural, maternally induced runt disease in a
human infant

Histoincompatibility and maternal immunologic status
influence trophoblastic invasion and placental size

Prevention of Rh isoimmunization in women at risk by passive
immunization with anti-D antibody

Presence of fetal erythrocytes in maternal circulation from 8th
week of gestation in man

Intrauterine fetal transfusion for treatment of erythroblastosis
fetalis

Resistance of trophoblast to transplantation immunity

1975

1970

1965

Production of mouse chimeras by zygote fusion—tetraparental or allophenic mice

Suggestion that sudden infant death syndrome (SIDS) is due to anaphylactic reactivity to aspirated cow's milk protein antigens

Evocation of HL-A antibodies in maternal serum by pregnancy

Attempted treatment of choriocarcinoma by maternal sensitization against husband's tissue antigens

Experimental procurement of GVH or runt disease in perinatal birds and mammals

Natural red cell chimerism in a human dizygotic twin

First systematic review of factors that might underlie success of fetus as an allograft

Rejection of skin allografts by fetal sheep of 100 days' gestation

Discovery of immunological tolerance

Mutual tolerance of dizygotic cattle twins to grafts of each other's skin

Natural red cell chimerism in dizygotic twin cattle

Maternal Rh isoimmunization due to fetal-maternal passage of erythrocytes

Toxemia of pregnancy an immunologically based disease?

Autoantigenicity of milk

Malignant melanoma of maternal origin in human infant

Non-antigenicity of trophoblast enables it to function as immunologic quarantining barrier?

Isohemagglutinins detected in secretions of the female reproductive tract

Recognition of fetus as allograft

Abortifacient activity of heterologous antiplacental serum

Autoantigenicity of spermatozoa and testicular homogenates

Belief that profligacy of women may lead to infertility

Choriocarcinoma: A tumor of fetal origin

Successful transfer of fertilized eggs in the rabbit

Natural and experimental transmission of immunity from mother to young via milk in mice

Recognition that maternal and fetal blood circulations are completely separate

1960
1955
1950
1940
1930
1900
1600

WITHDRAWN

THE

IMMUNOBIOLOGY

OF

MAMMALIAN
REPRODUCTION

ALAN E. BEER

RUPERT E. BILLINGHAM

Southwestern Medical School
The University of Texas Health Science Center at Dallas

PRENTICE-HALL, INC., *Englewood Cliffs, N.J.*

Library of Congress Cataloging in Publication Data

BEER, ALAN E (date)
    The immunobiology of mammalian reproduction.

    (Prentice-Hall foundations of immunology series)
    Includes bibliographies and index.
    1. Reproduction—Immunological aspects. 2. Preg-
nancy—Immunological aspects. 3. Mammals—Reproduction.
I. Billingham, Rupert E., joint author. II. Title.
[DNLM: 1. Reproduction. 2. Maternal-Fetal exchange.
3. Immunity. 4. Immunosuppression.   WQ205 B415i]
QP251.B38   599′.01′66   75-45089
ISBN 0-13-451666-4

© 1976 by PRENTICE-HALL, INC.
Englewood Cliffs, New Jersey

10   9   8   7   6   5   4   3   2   1

PRINTED IN THE UNITED STATES OF AMERICA

PRENTICE-HALL INTERNATIONAL, INC., *London*
PRENTICE-HALL OF AUSTRALIA PTY. LIMITED, *Sydney*
PRENTICE-HALL OF CANADA, LTD., *Toronto*
PRENTICE-HALL OF INDIA PRIVATE LIMITED, *New Delhi*
PRENTICE-HALL OF JAPAN, INC., *Tokyo*
PRENTICE-HALL OF SOUTHEAST ASIA PTE., LTD., *Singapore*

This book is dedicated to those lovable creatures who, unknowing of the principles of immunoregulation, benevolently sustained us and our children as allografts in utero, and to those who apply their skills to protect less fortunate individuals from the malice of immunologic disease before birth.

Foundations of Immunology Series

This series of monographs is intended to provide readers of diverse backgrounds with an authoritative and clear statement concerning significant aspects of immunology. Each volume represents an individual contribution by a distinguished scientist. As a series, they provide a comprehensive view of the field.

The editors have encouraged the individuality of each author in content and method of presentation. They have sought as the major objective of the series, that each monograph be comprehensible and of interest to a broad audience. The authors provide an authoritative treatment of important problems in major research areas, in which rapid development of new information requires an integrated and reliable evaluation. The series should therefore prove valuable to advanced college students, graduate students, medical students and house staff, practitioners of medicine, laboratory scientists, and teachers.

ABRAHAM G. OSLER
LEON WEISS

Contents

xi

Preface

Immunology intrudes into nearly every aspect of mammalian reproduction and affords an important means of analyzing or monitoring several of its components. The burgeoning interest in the immunobiology of tissue and organ transplantation witnessed by the past quarter century has provided a forceful stimulus to uncover the *modus operandi* of Nature's highly successful violation of the "laws of transplantation," expressed by the almost consistent delivery of live infants in outbred populations of mammals. Choriocarcinoma, a relatively uncommon tumor in Caucasians, has commanded an entirely disproportionate amount of attention, in terms of the literature and conference time devoted to it, as much because it is a highly successful fetal $\longrightarrow$ maternal allograft as because of its relatively high rate of spontaneous regression and susceptibility to chemotherapy.

Early studies on passive transfer of immunity from mother to offspring, i.e., the maternal immunologic endowment, on ovum transfer, on the development of alloantigens in fetuses, on the antigenicity of spermatozoa and testicular material, and on the antigenic relationships between placenta and kidney (like later investigations on Rh disease and its prophylaxis), and the ontogeny of the immune response have been pioneered and developed to a large extent by independent series of investigators who, for perfectly good reasons, saw no need to try to fit their various findings into an all-embracing or common framework.

Although there is no shortage of good reviews on many of these topics where immunology is very directly involved, there have been few attempts to produce a concise, general synthesis of the basic principles and concepts of the immunobiology of reproduction, its multiple origins, current controversies, unsolved problems, and future prospects and goals—clinical and experimental.

This volume represents an attempt to satisfy this need for the benefit of medical students; advanced students of developmental, reproductive, and immunobiology; and obstetrician-gynecologists, pediatricians, and perinatologists. The authors have assumed only a modest familiarity with the basic principles of general immunology and of reproductive biology on the part of the reader.

Limitations of space and the desire to produce an easily readable text have precluded assigning credit to many investigators whose contributions have been cited and synthesized. To them we tender our apologies and beg their indulgence. By way of compensation fairly extensive bibliographies have been provided at the end of each chapter to facilitate identification of our unsung heroes and, more important, to enable their contributions to be studied in extenso.

We are deeply indebted to our colleagues, especially to Dr. William B. Neaves for helpful criticism and suggestions, and to Mrs. Madelon Smith and Miss Trinidad Rubio for help with the manuscript, and to Mrs. Jean Billingham and Mrs. Kathy Grubbs for assistance with the illustrations.

It is a pleasure to acknowledge that our own research efforts and the gathering of the material for this book have been made possible largely by grants from the United States Public Health Service and the Lalor Foundation.

Dallas, Texas   ALAN E. BEER
                                                      RUPERT E. BILLINGHAM

Introduction

It is quite certain that man first became aware of the importance of immunology in mammalian reproductive biology unwittingly, through empirical observations on members of his own species as well as upon his domestic animals. For example, the Scriptures inform us that Sara, Abraham's first wife, was sterile for many years but eventually conceived. Dr. Seymour Katsh has suggested, possibly with tongue in cheek, that following her first coital exposures she became immunized to Abraham's seminal products. Then, during the long period of continence while Hagar was Abraham's second wife, Sara's immunity declined so that conception became possible.

The mutilating punishment prescribed by Assyrian laws for a woman who had crushed a man's testis in an affray took heed of the fact that after the damaged organ had been bound up by a physician, the second testis sometimes became affected. Here, again according to Katsh, what might have happened is that the initial injury released autoantigenic material, resulting in sensitivity that damaged the contralateral gonad. The frequent association of orchitis with mumps in mature but not in pre-pubertal males must also have been known from time immemorial, again probably reflecting the expression of an autoimmune response against an important component of the male reproductive system.

One can read into Charles Darwin's writings a connection between immunology and infertility. Like many of his contemporaries, he related the profligacy of women with reduced fertility. The possible inference here is that repeated exposure to antigenic material in the male ejaculate incited an immune response that resulted in sterility. It was probably this kind of reasoning that initiated a tremendous amount of work at the beginning of this century, and during the early days of immunology, on the antigenicity of spermatozoa, seminal plasma, and testicular preparations. This resulted in the classic independent publications of Landsteiner (1899), Metchnikoff (1900), and Metalnikoff (1900) that injections of sperm or testicular extracts into experimental animals led to antibody formation.

We can trace back to these early observations a long history of unsuccessful attempts, which still continue with increasing sophistication,

1

to devise an effective immunologic means of conception control in women based upon active sensitization to seminal antigens. From these early observations also stems the very plausible notion that some instances of sterility in apparently normal men and women may be the outcome of natural immunization to sperm-associated antigens. It is also pertinent to add that the recent tremendously increased application of vasectomy for male sterilization has occurred on the basis of a very inadequate knowledge of the possible long-term adverse immunologic consequences of the enforced retention of potentially autoantigenic material.

It is also interesting to recall at this juncture that in the 1920's Dr. F. R. Lillie advanced his classical *fertilizin* theory of fertilization based on the model afforded by the immunological knowledge of his day. He postulated that a sperm antigen, *antifertilizin,* plays an essential role in the sperm-egg interaction. Subsequent extensive studies by Dr. Albert Tyler, using rabbit antisera to sea urchin gametes, implicated the specific combining sites of sperm antigens in one or more essential steps in the fertilization of sea urchins.

Another immunologically based phenomenon associated with repro-duction with which man must have long been acquainted is hemolytic disease of the newborn infant, as well as that afflicting mule foals.

From the viewpoint of a transplantation immunologist mammalian reproductive activity affords certain gene products on cell surfaces, i.e., *transplantation* or *histocompatibility antigens* (in addition to certain tissue or cell-specific antigens)—opportunities to interact with immunologically competent cells in a variety of ways and at numerous sites. These are summarized in Fig. 0.1. There is (1) the repeated exposure or inocula-tion of female hosts, by one specific and highly specialized route, with hundreds of millions of highly specialized, motile, short-lived cells—spermatozoa of alien genetic origin—suspended in a complex protein-aceous medium; (2) the self-propulsion and dissemination of a significant proportion of this cellular inoculum along the female reproductive tract where it soon undergoes absorption and degradation by macrophage activity and other processes; (3) the fusion of a few of these cells, nor-mally on a one-to-one basis, with the much larger, free-floating ova to produce zygotes having equivalent genetic endowments from *both* parents; (4) these early conceptuses, after enjoying a "larval" type of existence of about 5 days' duration (in a few animals such as deer and the Euro-pean badger, which exhibit the phenomenon of delayed implantation, this may last for many months) subsequently engraft or implant themselves upon the endocrinologically prepared endometrial surface; (5) here, what is initially a simple, graft-host relationship matures into one that is more appropriately regarded as an intimate parabiotic union between genetically dissimilar organisms of disparate size and developmental status—the fetal-

NATURE AS A TRANSPLANTER

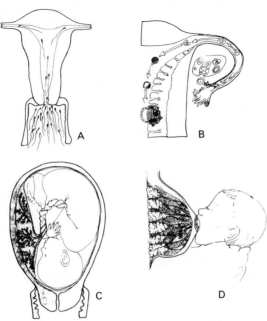

Fig. 0-1. Various events in mammalian reproduction involving transplantation. (A) Sexual inter-course, which culminates in the "inoculation" of the adult female hosts, via the intravaginal route, with cellular allografts comprised of large numbers of spermatozoa suspended in a complex medium, the seminal plasma. (B) Implantation, or engraftment, of the blastocyst upon the endocrinologically prepared endometrial surface of the uterus. (C) Development of the zygote reaches a stage when the maternal-fetal relationship is obviously a parabiotic union at the level of the placenta between two different organisms. Despite the invariable absence of anastomoses between the maternal and fetal blood circulations in this organ of physiologic exchange, covert cellular exchanges do occur. (D) After parturition, the breast takes over the nutritional and certain other roles from the placenta. Moreover, in some mammalian species viable leukocytes, which are normal ingredients of colostrum and milk, escape from the infant's gut gaining access to its bloodstream.

maternal relationship. An important distinction we must emphasize be-tween mothers and their fetuses as natural parabionts on the one hand and surgically produced parabionts on the other hand is the absolute *absence* of vascular intercommunications between the former. This, as we shall see, has both immunologic and physiologic significance. Gestation represents the duration of this fetal-maternal relationship that is of ap-proximately constant duration for any given species, ranging from 16 days in Syrian hamsters to 21 months in Indian elephants. It is important to emphasize the tremendous variation among species in the mean number of fetuses that normally develop concomitantly in the uterus, ranging from 1 in cattle and man to 10 or more in mice and rats (where at term collectively they may approach the maternal weight), and also in the total number of litters a female may give rise to during her reproductive life-span.

The fact that spermatozoa (1) possess built-in cytospecific antigens, in addition to (2) their recently established possession of transplantation antigens and (3) their natural propensity to absorb antigenic materials, including blood group substances, from the medium in which they are dispensed suggests the possible occurrence of one kind of maternal immunization or sensitization that might, either naturally or under experimentally procured conditions, interfere with the early stage of the reproductive process.

Studies on the fate of experimental and therapeutic grafts of tissues and organs exchanged between genetically dissimilar individuals have established the universality of the allograft reaction in untreated, immunologically mature hosts, highlighting the paradoxical normal success of the fetus as a genetically alien graft. This notion is sustained by the following empirical observations: (1) No progressive decline in fertility occurs with parity of a female by the same unrelated male. (2) Allografts from offspring resulting from such matings usually enjoy no special or significant dispensations when grafted to their mothers either during or after pregnancy. (3) It is exceedingly difficult, if not impossible, to cause mothers to reject immunogenetically alien fetuses by presensitization against the alien tissue transplantation antigens of their consorts. Great efforts have been stimulated on the part of both armchair theorists, as well as laboratory workers, to account for this consistently successful violation of the "laws" of transplantation. The paradox is heightened by evidence that, in an immunologic sense, mothers *are* aware of the presence of immunogenetically alien fetuses in their uteri and respond to them in a noncytopathogenic manner.

As we shall see, recent work indicates that being genetically disparate with regard to its mother—i.e., confronting her with alien transplantation antigens that sensitize her—confers a statistically significant selective advantage upon a zygote in two different ways: (1) It increases its chances of being implanted initially. (2) It results in increased placental and fetal growth.

It is ironical that those whose professional activity brings them most into contact with human fetuses—namely obstetrician-gynecologists—have until recently shown little awareness of and interest in the fact that the "allografts" they are concerned with thrive so well in untreated, nonimmunosuppressed, and potentially reactive hosts. In fairness to them, however, we must not neglect the fact that it was a member of their calling, James Blundell of Guy's Hospital in London, who in 1829 performed the first successful blood transfusion—a form of tissue transplantation—on a woman suffering from postpartum hemorrhage.

From the immunological point of view the maternal-fetal relationship is much more complex than the relationship between a tissue or an organ allograft and an immunologically mature host. This is a consequence of the fact that pregnancy entails a parabiotic union between two different *organisms* in which not only is there intimate apposition and commingling (at the trophoblast-endometrial interface) of relatively immobile tissue cells of genetically dissimilar genetic makeup but also, in some species, the fetal components of the placenta are constantly and directly exposed to host (i.e., maternal) blood as in the case of a renal allograft. In addition, there is evidence of a chronic, normally low-level, covert exchange of blood elements of various types between the maternal-fetal parabionts that has important potential, and in some instances very real, immunologic significance. For example, in the case of the offspring it may result in the development of a fatal wasting syndrome, known as runt or transplantation disease, due to graft-versus-host reactivity on the part of maternal lymphocytes that become incorporated in the tissues of the fetus.

The brilliant analysis of the etiology of hemolytic disease of the newborn in man by Stetson and Levine in 1938 indicated that the risks of isoimmunization through pregnancy (in this case as a consequence of the passage of fetal erythrocytes into the maternal circulation) are of more than academic interest—there are very definite immunologic hazards associated with being gestated. This work raises the possibility that other systems of isoantigens might also contribute to fetal mortality or morbidity. The highly successful *antibody-mediated* prophylaxis that has been developed for Rh-incompatible pregnancies at risk is a triumph of modern medical research and, at the same time, a source of encouragement that other untoward or harmful immunologic responses will indeed prove susceptible to control by simple, innocuous regimens.

The knowledge of the normal sensitization of the human mother to the antigens of her feto-placental unit is clearly important for the light it may shed upon the etiology of toxemia of pregnancy, a fairly common and still enigmatic disease that some workers believe has an immunologic basis. For example, McKay and his co-workers have likened this condition to a generalized Schwartzman reaction due to sensitization of the patient either to placental proteins or to a similar antigen, followed by a "shock" reaction precipitated by release of antigen possibly through premature placental separation or focal injury to the placenta.

Choriocarcinoma, a highly malignant tumor that is usually of trophoblastic and therefore of fetal origin (as opposed to the nongestational form of teratomatous origin), is unique in that it appears consistently to transcend histocompatibility barriers from fetus to mother with impunity. It merits our consideration for the light it sheds upon the biological properties of normal trophoblast and the possibility that it contains trophoblast-specific antigen(s) that may render it susceptible to immunotherapy. We shall also review evidence that normal trophoblast may have a similar, tissue-specific antigen(s)—i.e., an autoantigen(s) associated with it—and this might lend itself to clinical application as a means of terminating unwanted pregnancies at an early stage.

One of the classic, defining properties of an immunologic response is transferability of the reactivity from a putatively actively immunized subject to a normal, unimmunized subject, either by means of serum or by means of cells, depending on whether the immunity concerned is mediated by humoral antibodies or by cells of the lymphocytic series. Application of this principle to the prophylaxis and treatment of certain infectious diseases, notably tetanus and diphtheria, still occupies an important position in medicine despite the emergence of antibiotic therapy. Prophylactic immuno-therapy is an important principle, however, which evolved early in mammalian evolution, and the various means by which young mammals are enabled to enjoy most of the benefits of their mother's prior history of exposure to pathogens—via the so-called maternal immunologic endowment—is a fascinating and important component of our subject matter. The seemingly unassailable and widespread belief that the human infant acquires the totality of its useful quota of maternal antibodies across the placenta, *before* birth, has recently been shattered by the discovery of a new class of antibodies, IgA, which are unable to cross the placenta but are transmitted via the colostrum and milk. Although these antibodies are not absorbed from the infant's gastrointestinal tract, they do appear to exert an important protective effect within this milieu, especially against commonplace diarrhea-causing organisms.

The mammary gland and its exosecretions require our attention for a variety of reasons: (1) The breast manifests a highly selective uptake and secretion of certain antibodies from the maternal circulation. (2) IgA-type antibodies are synthesized locally within this organ in some species. (3) The exosecretion of these organs is not always beneficent. In some situations it can exert a harmful influence on the sucklings. For example, in mule foals suckled by mares, antibodies directed against donkey-specific erythrocyte antigens are absorbed via the gastrointestinal tract and cause a fatal hemolytic disease closely similar to erythroblastosis fetalis of man. (4) Milk contains at least one potentially autoantigenic ingredient, and a few cases of women becoming allergic to their own milk are on record so that the possibility of some infants becoming allergic to their mother's milk therefore exists. Allergy to milk from an unrelated species is a familiar, frequently distressing, and sometimes life-threatening event in human infants. Indeed, a strong case has been made that the "sudden infant death," or "crib death syndrome," has as its basis sensitization to allergens present in the formula diet.

Finally, viable leukocytes, including lymphocytes, at a concentration not greatly inferior to that of peripheral blood are a long-neglected but constant ingredient of colostrum and milk. In some species these cells enter the recipient's circulation where they may confer immunologic benefits—i.e., adoptive transfer of maternal cellular immunities. They can also elicit or induce transplantation immunity or tolerance with regard to maternal tissue antigens and cause graft-versus-host disease. Cogent grounds now exist for a revision of the tendency of modern society to dispense with breast feeding and regard it as an activity associated with peasants and barnyard animals.

The ontogeny of the capacity to react immunologically against antigens is another important facet of the immunobiology of mammalian reproduction. Work on this topic was stimulated by the concept of immunologic tolerance formulated by Burnet and Fenner in 1949 at a time when it was erroneously believed that fetuses were more or less immunologically incompetent, presumably because they develop in an environment that quarantines them from nearly all infectious microorganisms. It is very pertinent to mention that in formulating their theory of tolerance Burnet and Fenner were greatly influenced by Dr. Ray D. Owen's demonstration in 1945 that as a result of a natural prenatal exchange of erythrocyte precursors via anastomoses of blood vessels between the chorions of bovine twin embryos, most twin cattle are born with, and may retain throughout life, a stable though variable mixture of each others' erythrocytes—i.e., they are chimeras. Subsequently, as we shall see, this observation has been extended to other species, including marmosets and, very infrequently, man. Further stimulation of interest in the ontogeny of the immune response was afforded by the discovery of the role of the thymus about 15 years ago.

As Dr. W. R. Jones of the University of Sydney has pointed out, pregnancy in humans affords a valuable experimental model for the study of the etiology and pathogenesis of immunological diseases. This turns upon the fact that only one class of immunoglobulin, IgG, is transferred from the mother to the fetus via the placenta. For example, clinical observations suggested that neonatal thyrotoxicosis is a placentally transmitted maternal autoimmune disease. In adults serological manifestations of this disease include circulating antibodies against various components of the thyroid gland and a long-acting thyroid stimulator (L.A.T.S.) that is present in the gamma globulin fraction of most affected individuals. L.A.T.S. has the characteristics of an IgG autoantibody. The observation that there is a consistent association between the presence of L.A.T.S.

8 INTRODUCTION

in cord blood and the occurrence of passive neonatal thyrotoxicosis afforded a strong indication of a causal relationship between the two. In addition it helped confirm that L.A.T.S. is an etiologic agent in thyrotoxicosis.

This model has proved useful in animals too. For example, it has helped to establish that the thymus is the source of a humoral factor important in the maturation of the immune response. Mice thymectomized soon after birth have a diminished capacity to respond immunologically to certain particulate antigens and to skin allografts. Dr. David Osoba found, however, that pregnancy will induce a restoration of the immunological responsiveness of neonatally thymectomized female mice to sheep erythrocytes and skin allografts, almost certainly as a consequence of the transplacental passage into the maternal circulation of a humoral agent from the thymus glands of the developing fetuses.

REFERENCES

Darwin, C. 1898. *The descent of man and selection in relation to sex.* Appleton, New York.

Jones, W. R. 1971. "Human pregnancy—an experimental model for the study of immunological disease." *Aust. N. Z. J. Obstet. Gynaec.* 11:164–169.

Katsh, S. 1959. "Immunology, fertility, and infertility: a historical survey." *Am. J. Obstet. Gynecol.* 77:946–956.

Katsh, S. 1969. "Immunological aspects of reproduction." In *Ovum implantation* (M. C. Shelesnyak and G. J. Marcus, ed.). Gordon and Breach, New York, pp. 309–344.

McKay, D. G., Merrill, S. J., Weiner, A. E., Hertig, A. T., and Reid, D. E. 1953. "The pathologic anatomy of eclampsia, bilateral renal cortical necrosis, pituitary necrosis and other fatal complications of pregnancy and its possible relationship to the generalized Schwartzman phenomenon." *Am. J. Obstet. Gynecol.* 66:507–539.

Metz, C. B. 1972. "Effects of antibodies on gametes and fertilization." *Biol. Reprod.* 6:358–383.

Osoba, D. 1965. "Immune reactivity in mice thymectomized soon after birth: normal response after pregnancy." *Science* 147:298–299.

Singer, C., and Underwood, E. A. 1962. *A short history of medicine.* 2nd ed. Oxford University Press, London.

Tyler, A., and Brookbank, J. W. 1956. "Inhibition of division and development of sea urchin eggs by antisera against fertilizin." *Proc. Natl. Acad. Sci.* 42:308–313.

Chapter 1

Essentials of Reproductive Biology

The implantation of a fertilized ovum in the endometrium and its development and survival as a feto-placental unit for the duration of gestation reflects a highly successful solution of the problems attending the transplantation of one particular type of graft, the genetically alien fetal placenta, to one particular type of bed, the maternal uterus. The solution to the problems of establishing and maintaining the embryo within the uterus of mammals is obviously coeval with their origin and represents the complex coordinated development of their neurological, endocrinological, and immunological systems.

The feto-placental unit is an *allogeneic* transplant in every sense of the word (see Chapter 6). The essential hormonal, vascular and immuno-genetic parameters for the initial "healing-in" of the fertilized egg, its development into an organismic graft, and its ultimate and consistent "rejection" after a relatively constant survival time (gestation period) can be compared to those parameters pertaining to the initial acceptance and phase of functional well-being of the conventional grafts used in experimental immunobiology and replacement surgery.

With maturation of the hypothalamo-pituitary-ovarian axis of female mammals, cyclic physiologic processes are set in motion that prepare the reproductive organs for the event of pregnancy. The entire process is initiated by a series of molecular "messages" from specialized cells in the brain that activate neurosecretory cells in the hypothalamus to secrete gonadotropin-releasing hormones into the hypophyseal portal circulation whence they reach the pituitary gland. In response to these messages, endocrine cells of the pituitary release their stored supplies of luteinizing and follicle stimulating hormones (LH and FSH) into the general blood circulation. These hormones, working together, stimulate changes in the ovary that result in growth of ovarian follicles containing immature oocytes. During this maturation process, the oocytes enlarge rapidly; they resume their long-delayed meiotic activity, and the follicle cells surrounding these oocytes, apart from nourishing them, assume an endocrine role producing

9

ever-increasing amounts of estradiol. Ovulation of the mature oocytes is induced by a mid-cycle surge in the concentration of pituitary LH in the blood. Subsequently, the now empty follicle nest fills with blood and quickly transforms into a corpus luteum, a transient endocrine organ producing both estrogen and progesterone. These hormones unite to special receptors in the cells of the reproductive organs and stimulate their growth in preparation for pregnancy.

Each month the human female undergoes a physiological preparation for pregnancy. An oocyte is matured and ovulated; the tissues and secretions of the reproductive tract become receptive so that "inoculated" spermatozoa achieve safe passage to the oocyte; the secretory and muscular components of the fallopian tubes are prepared to nourish and transport the preimplantation zygote to the uterus at the appropriate time and, finally, the lining of the uterus is prepared to receive the blastocyst.

The events of this cycle remain unaltered until the blastocyst initiates its active incursion through the endometrial epithelium in search of a blood supply. If pregnancy does not ensue, the corpus luteum abruptly ceases to function and menstruation occurs. This cycle faithfully repeats itself monthly until no further oocytes remain in the ovary (menopause). These cyclic processes require an important part of the total energy produced by the individual but contribute very little to the total body economy.

PREIMPLANTATION STAGES OF PREGNANCY

After fertilization, which takes place in the mid-portion of the fallopian tube, the ovum invested and quarantined immunologically by the zona pellucida (see page 94), spends 3 or 4 days suspended in and nourished by the unique fluid secreted by the tubal epithelial cells. During this preimplantation sojourn it undergoes holoblastic cleavage, becoming a solid sphere of cells, and eventually develops into three layers. It is the repression and derepression of individual bits of genetic information at this early stage of development which results in the setting apart of the future primordial germ cells and the differentiation and organization of the somatic cells from the fetal trophoblast cells which completely invest the blastocyst. After a precisely timed interval the blastocyst, consisting of an embryonic pole of several dozen cells discretely separate from the trophoblastic elements of approximately several hundred cells, is delivered into the uterus where it remains free-floating until day 6 or 7 postfertilization when implantation is initiated.

In this environment, until its active invasion into the endometrial epithelium, the blastocyst imbibes its sustenance from the uterine glandular secretory products through the intact zona pellucida. Blastokinin, a low molecular weight protein secreted by the endometrial glands, induces and regulates development of the blastocyst prior to implantation. In the absence of this intrauterine protein, morulae arrest in the early stages of gastrulation, will not form a fully developed gastrocoele and will not implant. These observations provide an added indication of the unique parabiotic relationship between the graft and its host even *before* formal attachment is achieved. Dr. Beatrice Mintz of the Institute for Cancer Research in Philadelphia has shown conclusively in mice that, in addition to blastokinin, the uterus at the time of preimplantation pregnancy and as a result of higher hormonal control secretes a low molecular weight enzyme that specifically triggers the adhesion phase of the blastocyst with the endometrium and initiates lysis of the zona pellucida. She postulated that this enzyme, called *zonalysin,* directly or indirectly effects glycoprotein receptors on the surface of the blastocyst cells, causing them to become "electrostatically sticky," so initiating adhesion with the endometrial epithelial cells.

From fertilization to implantation the ovular and endometrial changes are closely coordinated and the success of implantation in the *endometrium* turns upon maintenance of this delicate synchrony. Like other tissue grafts, blastocysts are not very discriminating in terms of their requirements for implanting and developing more or less normally to a relatively advanced stage. This is evidenced by their performance when deliberately placed in such ectopic sites as the anterior chamber of the eye, the brain, the spleen, the cryptorchid testis, and the mesentery and by the fact that not infrequently they implant of their own accord and develop to an advanced stage in extrauterine sites such as the ovary, rectum, or pouch of Douglas in man. These organs are relatively insensitive to the hormones that stimulate the uterus and its epithelium.

By contrast, the endometrium, which is the natural recipient area for fertilized eggs, behaves in a much more discriminating manner. Not only is the phase during the reproductive cycle when it will accept blastocyst "grafts" sharply delineated but, despite the relatively enormous surface area of the endometrium available, there is a restricted distribution of potential implantation sites.

It is well established that the stage of maturation of the blastocyst is a critical determinant of its successful nidation. Utilizing blastocyst transfer techniques, it has been found by Doyle and his associates that ova younger than the appropriate stage of endometrial development fail to implant. The most favorable conditions in the reproductive cycle obtain when embryos are either in synchrony with or one day ahead of the endometrium. Dr. Anne McLaren has quite appropriately depicted the uterus as a Procrustean bed. An obvious structural feature that may contribute significantly to the discriminatory properties of the uterus as a recipient site in nonprimate species is its uninterrupted lining, throughout the reproductive cycle, by a layer of epithelium.

ROLE OF HORMONES IN IMPLANTATION

The receptivity of the uterus is under hormonal control. It has long been known that progesterone, produced by the developing corpus luteum in the ovary, prepares the estrogen-primed endometrium in a general way for implantation. In rats it has been shown that an estrogen surge on the fifth day of preimplantation pregnancy is essential for nidation to occur in the progesterone-primed uterus. This estrogen surge, of ovarian origin, is induced by pituitary gonadotropins under hypothalamic control. If the pituitary is removed, implantation does not take place unless exogenous progesterone and estrogen are administered. This complex endocrine control system is concerned entirely with the preparation of the uterus as a graft site, having nothing to do with the blastocyst's development.

ENDOMETRIAL-TROPHOBLASTIC RELATIONSHIPS AT IMPLANTATION

The epithelium of the uterine mucosa, just prior to implantation of the fertilized zygote, consists of two cell types: ciliated and nonciliated cells. Progesterone, secreted by the granulosa lutein cells of the corpus luteum following ovulation, causes a decrease in the numbers of ciliated cells. The nonciliated cells at the implantation site become multinucleated. Electron micrographs of the early contact stages show that the trophoblast of primates is syncytial at the time of attachment with the endometrium. At this stage, in some species, the endometrial epithelium at the implantation site is transformed into a symplasma—plasma membranes between individual cells disintegrate and the microvillous surface of the apical portions of the fused cells forms massive cytoplasmic processes that reach out into the uterine cavity and engage in an exaggerated endocytosis of macromolecules as well as particles. This symplasma change is dependent on the presence of the trophoblast and its enzymatic secretory products and does not occur during pseudopregnancy nor can it be induced by hormone treatment.

The syncytial trophoblast sends cytoplasmic processes into the nutritive milieu of the endometrial symplasma or between endometrial epithelial cells (see Fig. 1-1). In some species, large fetal syncytiotrophoblastic cell nuclei and smaller uterine epithelial cell nuclei become intermixed in a common cytoplasmic mass to which both mother and zygote have contributed. Indeed this process of "cell hybridization" is postulated to result in a living cytoplasm in which DNA, RNA, and cellular organelles of

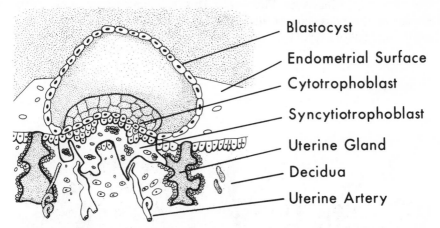

Blastocyst

Endometrial Surface

Cytotrophoblast

Syncytiotrophoblast

Uterine Gland

Decidua

Uterine Artery

Fig. 1-1. Diagramatic representation of a blastocyst of an 8-day human pregnancy in the process of implanting into the endocrinologically prepared endometrium. The uterine endometrium is richly vascularized at this time and the uterine glands are filled with nutritive glycogen-rich mucus. Note the multinucleated syncytiotrophoblast invading the uterine endometrial epithelium and the uterine glands and making initial contact with the maternal uterine arteries. By day 9 the blastocyst will be completely imbedded in the uterine endometrium. By day 11–12 the trophoblast will have eroded and migrated into the uterine vessels, exposing the alien tissue to maternal blood.

both maternal and zygote lineages are present. The only other recognized instance in which there is fusion of dissimilar cell types and sharing of dissimilar cell nuclei and cytoplasmic components occurs during the process of fertilization of an ovum by a spermatozoon. It has been suggested that this process of fusion of cytoplasmic elements of trophoblast and endometrium, which occurs prior to the penetration of the basement membrane of the uterine epithelium, may have immunologic significance in that the antigenic character of the resulting cells destined to invade the maternal blood vessels may be altered. No direct experimental confirmation of this seemingly attractive hypothesis has been forthcoming, however, and Drs. Gearhart and Mintz could find no evidence in the mouse that trophoblast cells incorporated maternal DNA. Following the embryo's adhesion with the endometrium, its distended blastocoele collapses, releasing its bicarbonate-rich fluid contents to the subjacent endometrium. The local influence of this fluid on the host tissue has been held responsible for the mobilization of maternally derived inflammatory and other cellular elements of hematogenous origin in the implantation site.

Following their penetration of the basement membrane of the uterine lining epithelium, the trophoblastic giant cells migrate deeply into the uterine endometrial stromal connective tissue and its underlying musculature where they are surrounded by plasma cells, mononuclear leukocytes, and macrophages of maternal origin for whose mobilization at the site they are responsible (see Fig. 1-2). This inflammatory reaction, reminiscent of the expression of allograft, tuberculin, and other types of cell-mediated, delayed-type hypersensitivities, promotes increased vascularity of the implantation site and brings to it a population of cells capable of removing the tissue and cellular debris resulting from the trophoblastic invasion. The end result of this "quasi-immunological" tissue response is the fully developed hypersecretory gestational endometrium (decidua) (Fig. 1-3). Besides initially satisfying the metabolic requirements of the

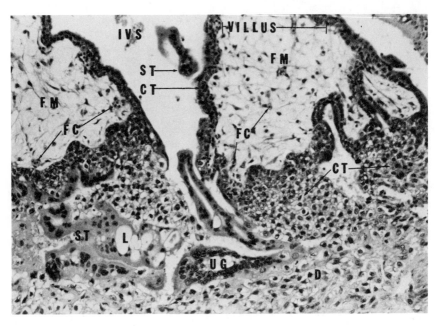

Fig. 1-2. Photomicrograph of a portion of the choriodecidual junction of a human conceptus of 8 weeks gestation. Maternal blood in the intervillus space (IVS) is in direct contact with the syncytiotrophoblast (ST) of the fetal villus. Multinucleate fragments of syncytiotrophoblast are shed into the maternal venous circulation from early in gestation. These viable cell clumps eventually lodge in the capillary network of the maternal lung where they undergo dissolution by processes thought not to involve immunological mechanisms. At this period of time during gestation the fetal mesenchyme (FM) of the villus is invaded by fetal capillaries (FC) and the fetal circulation to the villus is established. Nucleated fetal erythrocytes can be seen in the capillary lumens. The fetal villi are anchored to the uterine decidua (D) by columns of cytotrophoblast cells (CT). At this interface, involving tissues of differing genotypes, accumulations of small lymphocytes of maternal origin can be identified. Tongues of syncytiotrophoblast invade the uterine tissue more deeply, seeking the nutritive secretions of the uterine glands (UG). The island of syncytiotrophoblast to the left of the labeled uterine gland has formed large spaces called *lacunae* (L). These spaces become suffused with maternal blood once the trophoblast penetrates a maternal arteriole or vein. At parturition the placenta separates from the maternal decidua at the level of the cytotrophoblastic cell columns. Viable trophoblast can persist in the uterus for varying periods postpartum.

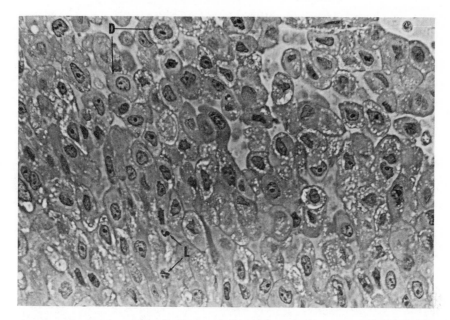

Fig. 1-3. Micrograph showing uterine decidual cells. Early in human gestation the fibroblast-like connective tissue cells of the uterine stroma undergo marked proliferative changes and assume an epithelioid appearance. These decidual cells (D), identifiable by their centrally located nucleus, which contains prominent nucleoli, are lipid and glycogen laden early in gestation. This succulent tissue milieu performs several functions: (1) It affords nutrition for the implanting conceptus. (2) It protects the uterus from whole-scale invasion by the trophoblast. (3) It may also afford a partial afferent lymphatic blockade preventing the entrance of trophoblastic tissue into draining maternal uterine lymphatics. In the vicinity of the invading trophoblast, "patrols" of maternal lymphoid cells (L) can be identified.

actively phagocytizing syncytiotrophoblast, this eventually limits the extent of its invasion of the uterine tissues.

Apart from engulfing erythrocytes and cellular debris of maternal origin, the phagocytic syncytial trophoblast actively takes up maternal plasma in the form of membrane-bound vesicles. Fluid trapped by this mechanism is utilized to supply constituents for the redistending blastocoele cavity. It may also transmit to the early embryo agents, including cells and viruses, that might be detrimental during early development.

By 8 days postimplantation the conceptus is completely buried in the uterine stromal connective tissue. Syncytial and cytotrophoblastic epithelium infiltrate the lush decidual tissue apparently "guided" or attracted to the spiral arteries in the superficial endometrium. Both syncytial and cytotrophoblast penetrate the vessel walls and begin to replace the native vascular endothelium. The internal elastic lamina of the vessel is invaded by trophoblast and round cells and the muscular tunica media is completely replaced by trophoblast. Thus the normally contractile uteroplacental arteries are transformed into noncontractile aneurysms. This physiological process serves to lower the peripheral resistance in the blood vessels supplying the intervillus space. The basal arteries located deeper in the uterine myometrium do not undergo these changes. Occasionally cytotrophoblast cells fill and occlude the uterine vessels and the syncytiotrophoblast cells extend for a considerable distance into the lumina of the spiral arterioles, migrating as far as the lumbar aorta in the human where they persist until the postpartum period. Once sufficient spiral arterioles have been opened by the invading syncytiotrophoblast, the lacunae within the trophoblast islands become suffused with maternal blood and the maternal circulation to the placenta, which by 20 weeks of pregnancy will reach ½ liter/min, is established.

Trophoblastic cells from an early stage in gestation onward are continuously being shed or exfoliated into the maternal venous circulation in numbers of the order of 100,000–200,000 cells/day. These eventually reach the lung where they undergo destruction by enzymatic processes unaccompanied by any demonstrable local host response, inflammatory or otherwise. The apparent inability of these ectopic trophoblastic grafts to proliferate and form benign metastases probably reflects their highly differentiated, end-cell status (see Chapter 6).

Once the maternal circulation to the placenta has been established, the fetal villi become highly branched and invaded by fetal mesenchyme and vessels. The fetal circulation is established 21 days postimplantation. The placenta villi continue to differentiate into longer and more highly branched structures through mitotic activity of the cytotrophoblast through the third month of gestation, exposing progressively greater areas of syncytiotrophoblast to maternal blood in the intervillous space (see Fig. 1-4). By the twentieth week of gestation the aggregate surface area of the fetal trophoblast in the human placenta is estimated to be 15 square meters.

It is certainly remarkable that the trophoblast in an ectopic site, such as the kidney, will invade *all* compartments of the organ, i.e., the tubules, glomeruli, arteries, veins, and lymphatics. In the uterus, by contrast, the orderly development of the decidua (see Chapter 2) presents a barrier of sorts to trophoblastic invasion. Although lymphatic vessels are abundant in the uterus, the developing decidual tissue effectively occludes these. It has been postulated that this process of decidualization affords an effective temporary afferent blockade preventing the immediate passage of placental and fetal subcellular or other antigenic material to seats of immunologic response in the host and possibly trophoblastic invasion of

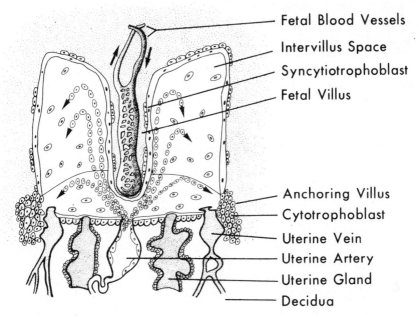

Fetal Blood Vessels
Intervillus Space
Syncytiotrophoblast
Fetal Villus

Anchoring Villus
Cytotrophoblast
Uterine Vein
Uterine Artery
Uterine Gland
Decidua

Fig. 1-4. A schematic representation of the mature human placenta, which is of the hemochorial type. The fetal tissue (chorion), consisting of three layers: syncytiotrophoblast, connective tissue, and vascular fetal endothelium, is in direct contact with maternal blood in the intervillous space. The cytotrophoblast of the anchoring villi is directly engrafted onto the maternal decidua. Fetal blood, rich in CO_2 and metabolic wastes of the fetus, is delivered to the placenta through the umbilical arteries, which repeatedly branch to supply the villi. Blood from the villi passes via a sinusoidal network into the umbilical vein, which carries oxygenated blood back to the fetus. The oxygenated maternal blood is delivered to the intervillous space by the uterine arteries, whence it spreads out in the intervillous space as depicted and circulates among the highly branched fetal villi. The venous blood returns via the uterine veins. Blood flow to the mature placenta is at the rate of about 500 ml/min.

their domain. Trophoblast cells have not been identified in the lymphatics draining the uterus of pregnant human subjects.

AN IMMUNOBIOLOGIST'S VIEW OF THE PLACENTA

The evolution of viviparity in vertebrates represents an exciting chapter in reproductive biology. As the higher forms evolved, quality not quantity became the central theme of reproduction. Offspring were fewer but bigger at delivery. To ensure the safe care and sustenance of these embryos the female of the species began to retain the fertilized eggs in the ovary or to transfer them to a brood pouch that represents a primitive type of uterus.

When the stored yolk of the fertilized egg was insufficient to nourish the developing embryo, ingenious parabiotic tissue unions developed between the mother and her fetus to serve as trophic or respiratory organs. As mammals appeared, the intimacy of the encounter between the maternal and fetal tissues increased and the trophoblast, a special mammalian adaptation to viviparity, appeared. It comprised the outer bounding layer of the fetal placenta across which all physiologic transactions between the parabionts had to take place. For the first time the uterus became an important organ. It developed into a temporary storage (halfway) house to see the embryo safely from the nourishing milieu of the ovarian follicle to the breast prepared to lactate. This successful intimate grafting of allogeneic fetal to maternal tissue took place despite the presence of a sophisticated immune system, which at first sight would appear to represent a built-in state of affairs destined to defeat this type of placentation.

Pregnancy in humans represents the highly developed end point of viviparous reproduction. The placenta of woman is an exceedingly complex organ comprised of tissues of two different genotypes. It must temporarily serve as a fetal lung, kidney, intestine, and liver as well as a complex endocrine organ that *completely* takes over the functions of the maternal ovary and pituitary and initiates and completes complex endocrine functions requiring input from both the mother and her immature fetus. In addition, the human placenta transmits to the fetus a dowry of prophylactic antibodies as it develops in a sterile environment, as if anticipating its sudden need of protection on exposure to the contaminated external environment at the time of parturition. None the less this relationship is always finite.

The placenta as seen in humans has pushed its parasitic parabiotic relationship with the maternal organism to *its ultimate*—its obligatory role, its treaty of compromise, is to preserve both the individuality of the mother as well as the fetus. If there were further invasion of the fetal trophoblastic epithelium, deeper into the maternal tissues, this could certainly result in the extinction of the species. We see the unfortunate results of the unchecked invasion of the trophoblast in man in the form of the malignancy, choriocarcinoma (see Chapter 7). This is a disorder in which the fetal trophoblast is not contained, invading beyond the uterine environment and metastasizing to vital organs such as the brain and lung. This unique tumor is almost universally fatal in untreated women despite its genetically alien status.

The placentas of mammals vary tremendously in their morphology. This situation is quite unique when compared to other organs of the fetuses of different species. For example, there is little structural variation in the liver, lung, kidney, and spleen. Nevertheless, the placenta, regardless of its structure, functions to bring the maternal bloodstream tenuously close to the fetal vessels and attempts to accomplish this task without allowing the cellular contents of the two compartments to mix. In man, unfortunately, this quarantine between the two vascular compartments is not completely efficient and the immunological consequences of the two-way leakage exchange of blood cellular elements in both the fetus and the mother have become evident in clinical medicine (see Chapter 11).

In order to understand more fully the human placentation it is helpful to look at the simplest form of mammalian placentation as seen in marsupials. Here the uterus merely serves as a shuttle path to bring the embryos from the nourishing milieu of the ovary to the breast in the pouch prepared to lactate. The placenta seems nothing more than a temporary compress against the uterine surface, where it remains attached for varying periods of time.

In this situation the uterine mucosa is apposed to the fetal membranes, collectively called the *chorion,* and the mucosa is never invaded or altered in the process. The fetal and maternal organisms are separated by six different tissue layers. In the human, as the placenta is developing early in pregnancy, one can follow histologically the appearance and subsequent erosion of most of these layers. As implantation progresses, there is a gradual breaking down of the barriers between the maternal and fetal blood compartments. The maternal tissue undergoes the greatest alterations. The chorion, or the fetal component of the placenta, remains relatively intact.

Further Notes About the Syncytial Trophoblast

All substances entering or leaving the fetal circulation must traverse the cytoplasm of the syncytial trophoblast (See Fig. 1-5). There are no intercellular spaces. This tissue is also the site of synthesis of the steroid and protein hormones in the placenta during gestation. HCG (human chorionic gonadotrophin) with similarities to pituitary LH and FSH and having a molecular weight of 59,000 is preferentially secreted into the maternal plasma. It is luteotrophic and is thought to stimulate placental steroid biogenesis by accelerating aromatization of neutral steroids, i.e., it accelerates the rate of conversion from androgenic hormones such as testosterone to estradiol. The syncytiotrophoblast also produces 250 mg of progesterone per day, 10 times the production rate of this hormone from the corpus luteum.

It is established that the fetal testis is well differentiated by the time the fetal pituitary begins to secrete LH. The suggestion has been made that HCG may stimulate testicular development in the absence of the fetal pituitary and serve an important role in sex differentiation.

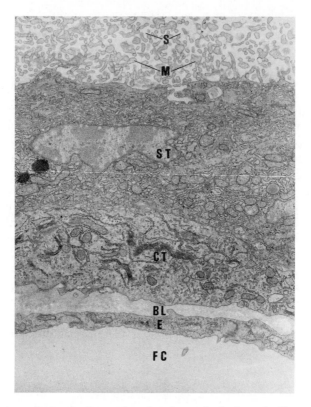

Fig. 1-5. Electron micrograph of a portion of a human fetal placental villus at 8 weeks of gestation. Maternal blood in the intervillous space (S) is in direct contact with the elaborate microvilli-covered surface (M) of the syncytiotrophoblast (ST). All substances from the maternal compartment entering the fetal circulation must traverse the syncytiotrophoblast (ST), the cytotrophoblast (CT), the apposed basal lamina (BL) of the cytotrophoblast and the fetal capillary endothelium, and finally the fetal capillary endothelium (E). The lumen of a fetal capillary (FC) has been sectioned longitudinally at the lower portion of this micrograph. Later in pregnancy, in the human, this "barrier" between maternal and fetal bloodstreams thins considerably in that the layer of cytotrophoblast cells disappears and the syncytiotrophoblast becomes much more attenuated.

Human chorionic somatomammotropin, sometimes referred to as human placental lactogen (HPL), which has both prolactin and growth hormone-like activity, is also secreted by the syncytiotrophoblast. This hormone has a glucose-sparing effect on the mother, directing glucose from the maternal metabolism toward that of the fetus since the entire energy source of the latter is glucose.

Human chorionic thyrotropin (HCT) is another syncytiotrophoblast hormone. It cross-reacts immunologically with thyroid-stimulating hormone (TSH) and may be essential for the early development of the fetal thyroid gland. Follicular development of the fetal thyroid begins at 8 weeks and iodination at 11 weeks, 3 weeks before fetal TSH production is initiated. The syncytiotrophoblast hormones discussed above are produced quite independently of the fetus. They appear in the maternal blood and urine in situations where viable trophoblast exists in the absence of a fetus. On the other hand, biosynthesis of estrogen by the syncytiotrophoblast requires combined efforts of both the fetus and the placenta since neither has the full range of enzymes required for the conversion of acetate or cholesterol to estrogen. It is well established that in women carrying anencephalic fetuses (these also lack the fetal zone of their adrenal cortex) the placenta produces little or no estrogen. This comes about because the fetal adrenal gland normally contributes a precursor that the placenta converts to estrogen(s).

REFERENCES

Beer, A. E., and Billingham, R. E. 1970. "Implantation, transplantation, and epithelial-mesenchymal relations in the rat's uterus." *J. Exp. Med.* **132**:721–736.

Beer, A. E., and Billingham, R. E. 1972. "Concerning the uterus as a graft site and the foetus as a natural parabiotic organismic homograft." Ontogeny of Acquired Immunity, Ciba Foundation Symp. *Elsevier Excerpta Medica,* North-Holland No. 5, 149–167.

Beier, H. N. 1968. "Uteroglobin: a hormone-sensitive endometrial protein involved in blastocyst development." *Biochem. Biophys. Acta.* **160**: 289–291.

Boyd, J. D., and Hamilton, W. J. 1970. *The human placenta.* Heffer, Cambridge, England.

Enders, A. C., and Nelson, M. 1974. "Pinocytotic activity of the uterus of the rat." *Am. J. Anatomy* **138**:277–300.

Gearhart, J. D., and Mintz, B. 1972. "Glucosephosphate isomerase subunit-reassociation tests for maternal-fetal and fetal-fetal cell fusion in the mouse placenta." *Developmental Biol.* **29**:55–64.

Kirby, D. R. S. 1970. "The egg and immunology." *Proc. Roy. Soc. Med.* **63**: 59–61.

McLaren, A., and Finn, C. A. 1967. "A study of the early stages of implantation in mice." *J. Reprod. Fert.* **13**:259–267.

Mintz, B. 1972. "Implantation-initiating factor from mouse uterus," In *Biology of mammalian fertilization and implantation* (K. S. Moghissi and E. S. E. Hafez, ed.). Charles C. Thomas, Springfield, Ill., pp. 343–356.

23 ESSENTIALS OF REPRODUCTIVE BIOLOGY

22   ESSENTIALS OF REPRODUCTIVE BIOLOGY

22 ESSENTIALS OF REPRODUCTIVE BIOLOGY

Moghissi, K. S. and Hafez, E. S. E., ed. 1974. *The placenta: biological and clinical aspects.* Charles C. Thomas, Springfield, Ill., p. 406.

Park, W. W., ed. 1965. *The early conceptus normal and abnormal.* D. C. Thomson and Co., Ltd., Dundee. Distributed by E. S. Livingstone Ltd., London, p. 147.

Parks, J. J., and Zimmer, F. 1973. "Immunologic aspects of the fetal-maternal relationship," in *Reproductive Biology* (H. Balin and S. Glasser, ed.). Excerpta Medica, Amsterdam, pp. 834–852.

Robertson, W. B., Brosens, I., and Dixon, H. G. 1967. "The pathological response of the vessels of the placental bed to hypertensive pregnancy." *J. Path. Bact.* **93**:581–592.

Segal, S. J. 1974. "The physiology of human reproduction." *Sci. Am.* **231**:52–62.

Chapter 2

The Uterus as a Graft Site

There are certain sites in the body that are known as immunologically privileged sites. These include the brain and the anterior chamber of the eye. In laboratory animals, the cheek pouch of the Syrian hamster is the best studied example. In these unique anatomical locations, tissue allografts can be grafted or implanted and, once vascularized, they survive for anomalously long periods of time seemingly exempt from immunologic rejection. In recent years Dr. Clyde Barker of the Surgery Department of the University of Pennsylvania has shown that immunologically privileged sites can be created surgically in rodents simply by excising a circular island of skin from its underlying connective tissue in such a way that a narrow central umbilical cord of connective tissue containing an artery and vein, but no lymphatic vessels, is preserved to nourish the uprooted skin flap. He demonstrated that skin allografts transplanted onto this island survive for many weeks, exempt from allograft rejection. The privileged status of the artificially created site, like that of the hamster's cheek pouch, turns upon the lack of afferent lymphatic pathways that connect with regional lymph nodes. These pathways are essential to convey antigenic material, or host lymphocytes that have been stimulated by antigen in the allograft, to a seat of immunologic response in the host. These privileged sites are totally unable to extend hospitality to the allografts they bear if the host is presensitized to the antigens concerned by prior exposure or is adoptively immunized during the course of the experiment. In these circumstances the blood vessels supplying the graft site convey sensitized lymphocytes to the foreign target.

For many years there has been the suspicion that the uterus might be an immunologically privileged site. Dr. Michael Schlesinger from The Hebrew University, Jerusalem, tested the possible privileged status of the uterus by implanting surgically, small tumor grafts into the uterine horns of rats and mice. He found that tumor grafts that were syngeneic with their hosts thrived in this milieu but that tumor allografts were rejected promptly in this site regardless of the endocrinologic status of the host, i.e., nonpregnant, normally pregnant, or pseudopregnant. Since some of the tumor allografts might have invaded beyond the physiologic boundaries of the uterine endometrium and entered adjacent tissue, it was impossible to deny a privileged status to the uterus on the basis of these experiments. It was subsequently demonstrated that allografts of normal, noninvasive tissue transplanted to the uterus under similar conditions described were consistently rejected. These findings suggested that transplantation immunity can be elicited as well as expressed in the uterus. The late David Kirby objected to these findings as decisively refuting the hypothesis that the uterus might be an immunologically privileged site, at least at the natural implantation sites of the allogeneic feto-placental units, for neither of the experimental "placebo" conceptuses described above incited a typical decidual response located in the uterus.

To investigate the possibility that the uterus might, under certain circumstances, be a privileged site required the introduction of tissue or cellular allografts as model conceptuses into the intact uterine lumen under atraumatic conditions that would prove conducive to their natural implantation. It was found that small skin grafts or suspensions of skin epidermal cells introduced into the uterine lumen healed-in consistently and very readily on the untraumatized endometrium, provided that the endometrium was in the proliferative phase and the host animal had not ovulated. Contrary to expectation, no decidual response was elicited in the uterus. In this anatomically unnatural site, genetically compatible grafts of skin or skin cells survived indefinitely, but when the intrauterine skin grafts were from genetically alien donors, they incited and succumbed to typical allograft reactions, surviving no longer than they would have done if transplanted orthotopically. Under conditions of the grafting described, the nonpregnant uterus affords no more hospitality to a skin allograft than does a conventional site prepared in the integument.

If host female rats are in the preimplantation stage of pregnancy or are made pseudopregnant by appropriate mechanical stimulation of the cervix at the time of insertion of skin allografts into their uteri, typical decidual responses consistently develop beneath these grafts. Under these experimental conditions the survival of the skin allografts was significantly prolonged. These findings support Kirby's idea that the decidual tissue that develops at the site of implantation of the conceptus might afford some immunologic protection to the fetal allograft. The possibility that the increased life-span resulted from a nonspecific, hormone-mediated suppression of the host's response was refuted by the observation that skin allografts transplanted to conventional sites on pregnant or pseudopregnant hosts were rejected with normal promptitude.

Unlike the situation with primary or first-set skin allografts in immunologically virgin hosts, decidual tissue afforded no protection whatsoever to intrauterine skin allografts placed in the uteri of specifically presensitized hosts. Here rejection of the grafts took place so rapidly that they failed to heal in properly.

These findings are consistent with the conclusion that decidual tissue subjacent to the alien skin graft in nonimmune subjects affords a partial blockage of the afferent lymphatic vessels. This blockade may prevent foreign antigenic material from reaching the proximal seat of immunologic response in the host—the regional para-aortic lymph nodes—or it may interrupt the passage of "peripherally" sensitized maternal lymphocytes to these organs. Another possibility is that this lymphatic obstruction facilitates the presentation of fetal antigenic material by the intravenous route, which is known to favor the development of enhancing or "blocking" antibodies capable of frustrating both the development and the fulfillment of cellular immunity (see Chapter 3). Suggestive evidence that decidual tissue can indeed afford the early conceptus some degree of immunologic protection is provided by Simmon's and Russell's demonstration of the vulnerability of early allogeneic zygotes placed in decidual-deficient ectopic locations, in preimmunized hosts, which is in contrast to their invulnerability in the uterus.

Elicitation and Expression of Immunity in the Uterus

When allografts are transplanted to most sites in the body, or suspensions of allogeneic cells are injected into tissues, there soon follows the hypertrophy of the regional lymph nodes draining the graft site. This is an indication that immunologically competent cells within these organs have been stimulated by alloantigens of the graft and that these stimulated cells engage in proliferative and other events that underlie the immune response.

When skin allografts or suspensions of allogeneic epidermal cells, leukocytes, or spermatozoa are inoculated directly into the uterine cavity, they incite a very significant enlargement of the lymph nodes draining this organ—the para-aortic nodes—and a state of transplantation immunity in the host (see Figs. 2-1, 2-2, and 2-3). This suggests that these draining nodes are the main site of the host's reactivity against the intra-uterine graft and that antigenic material in the uterine cavity is able to cross its endometrial lining and enter the lymphatic vessels of the organ.

Washed epididymal spermatozoa inoculated directly into the uterus of rats, mice, and hamsters, although slightly inferior to lymph node cells from the viewpoint of their capacity to incite transplantation immunity, are not inferior incitors of lymph node enlargement. Dosages of epididymal

Procedure for injecting cell suspensions
into uterine lumen

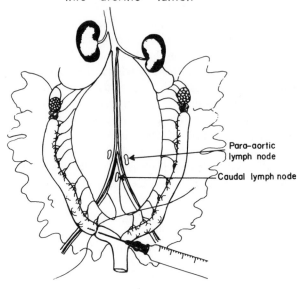

Para–aortic
lymph node

Caudal lymph node

Fig. 2-1. Illustrating the highly vascular bicornuate uterus of a rat, with its associated and neighboring structures. These include the ovaries with their convoluted fallopian tubes, the kidneys, the dorsal aorta and inferior vena cava, and the paired para-aortic lymph nodes, each of which drains the ipsilateral uterine horn. Inoculation of cell suspensions into the uterine lumen is easily accomplished by the technique illustrated after surgical mobilization of the organ. A fine soluble ligature is necessary to prevent the inoculum from draining away via the vagina. After the suture material has dissolved, however, patency returns and normal pregnancies can occur in a previously inoculated uterine horn.

spermatozoa that evoked transplantation immunity in the host, when inoculated by the intrauterine route, were totally ineffective when inoculated into the foot pads of the host. These findings sustain the view that contaminating leukocytes or other cells in the sperm inocula were not responsible for the immunity elicited and raised intriguing questions concerning the mechanisms whereby sensitization via the intrauterine route was achieved (see Chapter 5). Do these highly specialized cells traverse the uterine epithelium in sufficient numbers and bring their individual minute quotas of antigen directly to bear in the host tissue, possibly in the draining nodes, or are they taken up from the lumen by macrophages that act as both processors and transporters of the antigen? Evidence that epididymal spermatozoa are antigenically much more effective when inoculated into the uterus than into other sites hints that some special immunologic transaction may occur in this organ. It is quite possible that somatic fertilization of considerable numbers of endometrial epithelial cells occurs, followed by synthesis within them of alloantigens of the

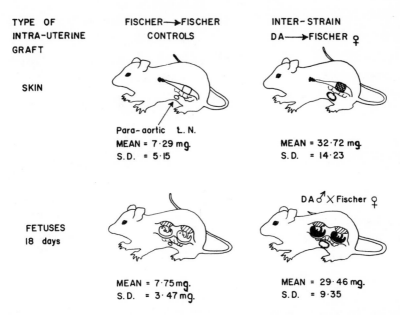

TYPE OF
INTRA-UTERINE
GRAFT

FISCHER→FISCHER
CONTROLS

INTER-STRAIN
DA———➤FISCHER ♀

SKIN

Para-aortic L. N.
MEAN = 7·29 mg.
S.D. = 5·15

MEAN = 32·72 mg.
S.D. = 14·23

FETUSES
18 days

DA ♂ X Fischer ♀

MEAN = 7·75mg.
S.D. = 3·47 mg.

MEAN = 29·46 mg.
S.D. = 9·35

Fig. 2-2. Influence of the presence of allogeneic skin grafts or fetuses in the uteri of female Fischer rats on the weight of the draining, para-aortic lymph nodes. The presence of DA skin allografts or of (Fischer × DA)F_1 hybrid fetuses in the uterine horns incite a specific, approximately fourfold, increase in the weight of the draining para-aortic lymph node about 10 days after grafting or conception.

donor type. This certainly would constitute an antigen-amplifying mechanism for nondividing spermatozoa.

Allogeneic spermatozoa deposited normally into the mouse uterus during coitus also induce hypertrophy and hyperplasia in the para-aortic nodes; however, in this circumstance they, dispensed in seminal plasma, are unable to incite a generalized state of immunity in the female.

Similar striking hypertrophy of the nodes draining the uterus can be observed in pregnant rats, mice, hamsters, and women bearing genetically alien fetuses; whereas much less significant enlargement of the nodes is associated with the presence of syngeneic fetuses (see Fig. 2-2). The only reasonable interpretation of these findings is that tissue alloantigens of fetal origin find their way into the draining maternal uterine lymphatics and stimulate the enlargement. Allogeneic fetuses, despite their ability to stimulate the regional lymph nodes, do not increase the host's resistance to test tissue allografts: Indeed, they seem to weaken it. This is thought to be due to their ability to evoke the formation of humoral antibodies corresponding to the major unshared histocompatibility determinants of their progeny. Whatever their significance, these responses have no ad-

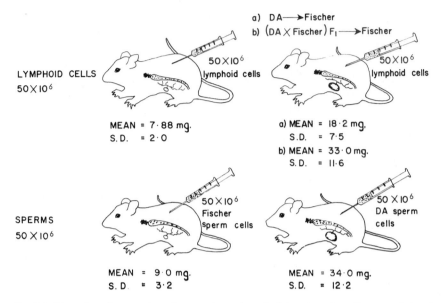

Fig. 2-3. Illustrating the capacity of suspensions of washed lymph node cells or epididymal spermatozoa from allogeneic DA strain donors inoculated into the uterine lumen of Fischer female rats to incite a striking, specific hypertrophy of the draining para-aortic lymph node.

verse effect on the fetus. In fact, there is evidence that they may even be beneficial to its development.

RECALL-FLARE REACTIONS IN THE LOCALLY SENSITIZED UTERUS

Following primary immunization of female rats against tissue antigens of an allogeneic donor strain by means of an intrauterine skin graft as described above or by means of an intrauterine inoculum of a viable suspension of allogeneic cells—they may be epidermal cells, spleen cells, lymph node cells, or washed epididymal spermatozoa—the uterus acquires the long-persisting capacity to respond to local reexposure or challenge with the same cellular antigen by a striking reaction. After a delay of 24–48 hours the challenged uterus becomes conspicuously inflamed and edematous, its tissue infiltrated by leukocytes, and its lumen dilated as a consequence of the buildup of fluid (see Fig. 2-4). This reaction subsides and the organ reassumes its normal appearance, both to outward inspection and histologic examination, within 4 days. This striking response, incitable in the locally sensitized uterus, cannot be evoked by challenge inoculation of the uteri of females presensitized against the same alien tissue antigens

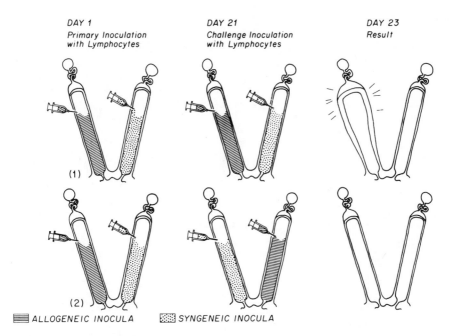

DAY 1
Primary Inoculation
with Lymphocytes

DAY 21
Challenge Inoculation
with Lymphocytes

DAY 23
Result

(1)

(2)

▤ ALLOGENEIC INOCULA   ▥ SYNGENEIC INOCULA

Fig. 2-4. The recall-flare reaction to tissue antigens in the rodent uterus. Female rats of one strain were inoculated in their right uterine horns with a suspension of viable allogeneic lymphoid or epidermal cells or washed spermatozoa prepared from the epididymis and in their left uterine horns with a similar suspension of cells of syngeneic origin. This procedure was repeated 21 days later; however, some of the animals received the allogeneic cells in their right uterine horns and syngeneic cells in their left uteri as before, and in others the delivery of the two types of secondary inocula was reversed. After a delay of 24–48 hours, the uterine horns that had been both primed and subsequently challenged with the alien cells developed striking recall-flare reactions, becoming transiently inflamed and swollen. When the priming inoculum of alien cells had been delivered into one uterine horn and the secondary, challenge inoculum of alien cells was administered into the opposite horn, however, no reaction was incited, indicating persistence of the hyperreactivity induced by the primary inoculum on a very local basis.

by any other route. For example, an orthotopic skin allograft is completely ineffective in this respect. Furthermore, a female rat that has been immunized locally in one uterine horn fails to give a local response if the challenge inoculum is subsequently introduced into the contralateral, nonlocally immunized uterine horn or intravenously (Fig. 2-5).

If a female, which has been subject to local intrauterine sensitization against the tissue antigens of an alien donor rat strain, is subsequently mated to a male of that strain, this local hypersensitivity reaction also manifests itself. Here spermatozoa in the ejaculate passing into the locally presensitized uterine horn presumably furnish the challenge inoculum (see Fig. 2-6).

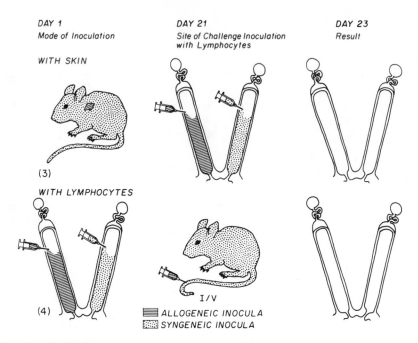

DAY 1
Mode of Inoculation

DAY 21
Site of Challenge Inoculation
with Lymphocytes

DAY 23
Result

WITH SKIN

(3)

WITH LYMPHOCYTES

(4)

I/V

▤ ALLOGENEIC INOCULA
▩ SYNGENEIC INOCULA

Fig. 2-5. Evidence that recall-flare reactivity is only incitable in animals sensitized by the intra-uterine route and challenged by this route. To generate the hypersensitive state revealed by the uterine recall-flare reaction sensitization by the uterine route appears to be mandatory. An orthotopic skin allograft is ineffective, though an intrauterine skin allograft is just as effective as an inoculum of allogeneic cells. Furthermore, animals that have received a primary inoculum of allogeneic cells in the lumen of their uterus fail to develop reactions in these organs if the challenge inoculum is delivered by the intravenous route.

This local, "recall-flare" reaction within the uterus is believed to be an expression of the reactivation of relatively small numbers of dormant host immunological "memory" cells that persist within the uterine mucosa and stroma long after the initial intrauterine sensitization.

INFLUENCE OF LOCAL SENSITIZATION OF THE UTERUS ON ITS SUBSEQUENT REPRODUCTIVE PERFORMANCE

The fact that the recall-flare reaction is readily incitable in the locally sensitized uterus by various types of monodisperse suspensions of viable allogeneic cells, including spermatozoa provided during normal mating, raised the interesting question whether it might be incited by or exert any discernible influence upon either the implantation or the subsequent development of F_1 hybrid conceptuses resulting from matings between females with locally sensitized uteri and allogeneic males against whose tissue antigens the sensitivity was directed.

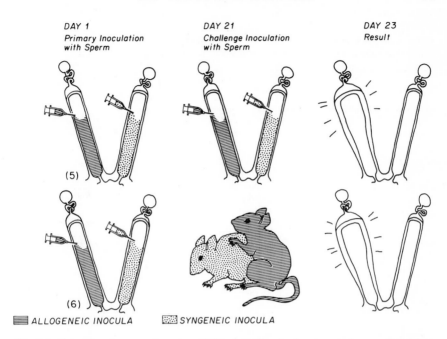

DAY 1
Primary Inoculation
with Sperm

DAY 21
Challenge Inoculation
with Sperm

DAY 23
Result

(5)

(6)

▤ ALLOGENEIC INOCULA   ▦ SYNGENEIC INOCULA

Fig. 2-6. Illustrating the evocation of recall-flare reactions in female rats by experimental or natural inoculation of allogeneic spermatozoa from an alien donor strain into the uterine horns of rats locally presensitized by inoculation of washed epididymal spermatozoa.

Experiments were conducted in which panels of virgin female rats were immunized in one uterine horn by means of skin allografts from donors of a genetically unrelated strain. Three weeks later, when local hypersensitivity was demonstrable, they were mated with males of the strain against whose tissue antigens the sensitivity was directed or with males of their own strain. Comparison of the number of fetuses which developed in the locally immunized uterine horn with the number which developed in the contralateral nonimmunized horn or in the uterine horns of unimmunized control animals revealed that prior local immunization significantly *increased* the reproductive efficiency of the organ (see Table 2-1). It was also found that the feto-placental units within the locally immunized uterine horns were heavier than their counterparts in their nonimmune homologues. It soon became apparent that this advantage must have an immunologic basis since it did not apply to genetically compatible conceptuses in uterine horns sensitized against the tissue antigens of rats of an unrelated third-party strain.

These findings, as well as the others presented or reviewed above, indicate that the uterus is (1) a very efficient route for the initiation of transplantation immunity both by solid tissue allografts as well as by viable monodisperse suspensions of cells and (2) able to express a state

Table 2-1

Influence of local presensitization of rat's uterus against alloantigens of subsequent fetuses on its reproductive performance

Number of FI females studied	Source of skin allografts used for local intrauterine immunization	Paternal strain	No. of fetuses in locally immunized uterus and no. of fetuses in unimmunized uterus	Mean litter size per uterus
13	LE	LE	63/47	4.8 ± 1.5
				P < 0.01
				3.6 ± 0.8
8	LE	FI (specificity control)	36/38	4.5 ± 1.8
				4.7 ± 1.8
11	DA	DA	56/36	5.09 ± 2.2
				P < 0.05
				3.2 ± 2.4
9	DA	FI (specificity control)	30/29	3.3 ± 1.6
				3.2 ± 1.3

Four panels of Fischer (FI) strain female rats were immunized locally in their right uterine horns by means of skin allografts from Lewis (LE) or DA strain donors. Three weeks later, when intense local hypersensitivity reactions were known consistently to be incitable by cellular inocula from the original donor strain, panels of these animals were mated with Lewis, Fischer, or DA males. At 18 days' gestation, the pregnant females were killed and the number of conceptuses in the locally presensitized (right) and the untreated uterine horns (control) were counted separately. The results presented in the table show very clearly that significantly more blasto-cysts implanted and developed in uterine horns in which they were capable of eliciting local reactions against paternally inherited alloantigens than in horns in which they were incapable of doing so.

of immunity as effectively as any other site in the body. Paradoxically, the immunogenetically alien feto-placental unit in this environment is completely undaunted. Its success most likely reflects the capacity of the trophoblast to function as an antigenically neutral buffer zone on behalf of the fetus, preventing host lymphocytes from engaging with fetal cells in a manner that will lead to transplantation immunity as well as pre-venting lymphocytic effector cells from a sensitized female from harming vulnerable fetal cells at the level of the placenta (see Chapter 6). This interpretation is consistent with that of Kirby who demonstrated that pre-implantation zygotes more disparate with their mothers at certain histo-compatibility loci were implanted with greater frequency than those less disparate. In addition he showed that decreasing the mother's ability to respond immunologically to the alien antigens of the blastocyst, by employing immunosuppressive procedures, resulted in a marked decrease in the number of conceptuses implanted. Observations such as these afford no grounds for the belief that a feasible means of conception control can be based upon transplantation antigens.

GRAFT-VERSUS-HOST REACTIVITY IN THE UTERUS

The various experiments cited so far strongly indicate that lymphoid cells introduced into the uterine lumen traverse the endometrial epithelium and reach the draining para-aortic lymph nodes. The possibility of inciting local, graft-versus-host (GVH) reactions in the uteri of F_1 hybrid hosts by inoculation of lymphoid cell suspensions from parental strain donors was explored in our laboratories. It was found that the uteri of hybrid females that were inoculated with suspensions of lymph node cells from parental strain donors became strikingly enlarged, edematous, and fluid-filled. The reaction reached its acme at about 48 hours postinjection. This uterine reaction was followed by a very rapid enlargement and increase in cellularity of the para-aortic nodes. A progressive increase in the node weight occurred from the second day onward until at least the ninth day postinoculation. It was found that the para-aortic node assay for GVH reactivity was just as sensitive and possibly more so than the currently used popliteal node assay in which the cells under study are inoculated into the foot pad, despite the fact that with the former the cells must find their own way from the uterine lumen across the endometrial epithelium to gain access to a draining lymphatic system.

Overtly this GVH reactivity closely resembled the recall-flare reactivity evokable in the presensitized uterus. Uteri that had been the sites of GVH reactivity soon underwent an irreversible atrophy, however, and behaved as if permanently incapable of sustaining further pregnancies. F_1 hybrid females that had sustained GVH reactions in both uterine horns subsequently mated normally but never became pregnant.

REACTIVITY OF FETUSES AGAINST THEIR MOTHERS

Since as we've already seen, (1) lymphoid cells deposited in the uterine lumen of a rat can easily traverse the intact endometrial epithelium and apparently gain access to the regional nodes, (2) it is reasonably well established that rats and mice acquire the capacity to react against some transplantation antigens before birth, and (3) there is evidence that the murine placenta contains immunocompetent cells of fetal origin, it seemed possible that, in situations where fetuses are sustained by genetically tolerant F_1 hybrid mothers and against some of whose antigens they are capable of reacting immunologically by virtue of their own genetic constitution, natural passage of fetal immunologically competent cells into maternal tissue might initiate graft-versus-host reactions that would reveal themselves locally in terms of hypertrophy of the draining para-aortic nodes draining this organ.

For example, if (Lewis × BN)F_1 hybrid female rats (AgB^1/AgB^3) are backcrossed to BN males (AgB^3/AgB^3), the females have all the genetic determinants of the transplantation antigens of both of their paternal strains and are consequently genetically tolerant of and incapable of mounting an immunologic attack against any of the cellular antigens of their R_2 backcross progeny. Some of the latter, however, should be capable of reacting against some of their mother's histocompatibility antigens as a consequence of their failure to inherit certain Lewis strain histocompatibility genes from them. For example, the Ag-B genotype of 50% of the progeny should be Ag-B^3/AgB^3 and these animals should be capable of reacting against the strong AgB^1 antigen present on the maternal cells.

We have tested this possibility in rats, mice, and hamsters by setting up appropriate matings. The experiments in all three species show very clearly that the presence of backcross fetuses in the uterus does lead to a significant increase in the weight as well as the cellularity of the maternal para-aortic nodes as determined during the latter part of gestation. The most reasonable interpretation of these findings is that the observed enlargement of the maternal regional nodes is an expression of graft-versus-host reactivity. An alternative explanation is that it reflects stimulation of these nodes by fetal antigens. The fact that only a slight increase in node size was observed in females bearing syngeneic fetuses militates against such a possibility.

IMMUNOGENETIC ASPECTS OF IMPLANTATION, PLACENTATION, AND FETO-PLACENTAL GROWTH RATES

When animals of two different inbred strains are mated, so that the F_1 hybrid embryos resulting confront their mothers with alien paternally inherited histocompatibility antigens, the litters tend to be larger and healthier than those resulting from intrastrain matings. It is commonly asserted that this disparity is due to heterosis or to hybrid vigor. The observations provide no hint, however, as to the nature of the mechanism(s) contributing to more and bigger feto-placental units. Does the status of a mother's immunological reactivity toward the alien tissue antigens of her conceptuses make any significant contribution to either the weight of the placenta or of the fetus associated with it?

Immunologically Based Conditioning of the Uterus
Procured by Allogeneic Matings

We have determined that a single natural intrauterine exposure of virgin mice to spermatozoa from males of an allogeneic strain incites a twofold to threefold increase in weight of the regional lymph nodes draining the uteri of virgin, tubal-ligated recipients. The peak reactivity of this immunologic response of the female host occurred locally at 4-5 days after a successful mating, a time when the blastocysts normally would present themselves to the uterine endometrium. This observation suggested that at this time the uterus itself might be hypersensitive or reactive and that this might make some contribution to the hospitality that it extends differentially to histoincompatible embryos.

Appropriately designed experiments undertaken to test this premise in some srains of mice, rats, and hamsters showed that semiallogeneic litters, i.e., F_1 hybrids, were significantly larger than genetically compatible ones, and in various strains of mice tested there appeared to be a causal relationship between the fetal-maternal incompatibility (which incites the harmless immunologic response of females to the allogeneic fetuses in their uteri) and this augmented incidence of implantation. Female mice, which prior to mating had been rendered specifically tolerant or unresponsive to tissue antigens of an alien strain and then mated with males of this strain, produced significantly smaller F_1 hybrid litters than normally reactive females mated with the same allogeneic males. Systemic sensitization of females to paternal antigens prior to mating did not further increase litter size above that seen in normal females.

Drs. Finkel and Lilly (1973) made similar observations in mice. They showed that there was a tendency for increased numbers of implantations per litter with increasing histoincompatibility between the mothers and their fetuses. They concluded that this may confer the histoincompatible fetus with a selective prenatal survival advantage.

Two other independent studies, by Michie and Anderson in 1966 and by Palm in 1970 and 1974, also have furnished strong evidence of the operation of histocompatibility gene-based selective pressures that assure the survival of excess numbers of heterozygotes (see Chapter 15).

Histoincompatibility and Maternal Immunologic Status as Determinants of the Size of the Feto-Placental Unit

In 1964 Dr. W. D. Billington made the interesting observation in mice that $(C57 \times A_2G)F_1$ hybrid fetuses, differing from their C57 mothers at the important H-2 locus as well as other H loci, had significantly heavier placentas than did homozygous fetuses of either parental strain. Comparison of the size of placentas from intrastrain C57 matings with those that developed when fertilized eggs from such matings were transferred to the uteri of H-2 locus incompatible A_2G strain surrogate mothers dismissed the obvious possibility that hybrid vigor was solely responsible. These observations were subsequently confirmed by James.

To evaluate the influence of fetal-maternal incompatibility on the invasive properties of trophoblast uncomplicated by the uterine milieu with its inevitable decidual response, Billington (1965) subsequently transplanted ectoplacental cones from 7½ day murine embryos to the testes of adult hosts. These grafts produced luxuriant growths of trophoblast. When the ectoplacental cones were transplanted to H-2 incompatible hosts, the extent of trophoblastic invasion proved to be even greater than when transplanted to syngeneic hosts.

Subsequent studies by James confirmed that this phenomenon had an immunogenetic basis. He demonstrated that the immunologic status of the mother with regard to the alien tissue antigens of her fetus was an important determinant of placental size and the growth of the fetus. In C57 mothers presensitized against A_2G tissue antigens, $(C57 \times A_2G)F_1$ hybrid fetuses developed significantly larger placentas than similar fetuses born by normal mothers. Furthermore, the placentas of similar F_1 hybrid fetuses borne by mothers that had been rendered tolerant of the antigens of the A_2G strain were significantly smaller than those of normal, untreated mothers. These important observations indicated that immunologic reactivity on the part of the mother was in some way responsible for placental size. Histological studies suggested that the increased placental weights attributable to immunological factors might be due to incorporation of more decidual tissue in the placenta but left open the question of whether more extensive trophoblastic invasion was involved.

Dr. Anne Clarke, on the other hand, working with mouse strains identical to those used by Billington and James, was unable to show that placental size was increased when C57BL females were immunized prior to mating with A_2G or CBA males. She states that in each of her experiments specific immunization had no effect on placental growth, but it did reduce fetal growth. These interesting findings merit confirmation in the rat.

These findings pose many interesting questions, some of which will be formulated and answered in the following paragraphs:

1. Do genetic disparities not involving the H-2 locus cause placental enlargement? Studies conducted on pregnant C3H females bearing fetuses with CBA strain alloantigens showed that allogeneic placentas in normal females are significantly heavier than syngeneic placentas and that a state of immunologic tolerance in the mother results in a decrease in placental

weight. In this instance the placentas of tolerant mothers were still heavier than those in syngeneic pregnancies and presensitization of the mothers did not result in heavier placentas.

In reciprocal experiments to analyze the influence of the immunological reactive status of female mice on their H-2 compatible allogeneic fetuses it was found that CBA females bearing (CBA × C3H)F_1 hybrid fetuses produced heavier hybrid feto-placental units than CBA females bearing syngeneic feto-placental units. Immunologically tolerant mothers produced placentas whose mean weight was essentially similar to that of syngeneic placentas. At least in these H-2 compatible female-male combinations there is evidence that genetic disparities not involving the H-2 locus do cause placental enlargement.

2. Does the principle apply to species other than mice, rats, and hamsters? A report by Hancock and his associates in 1968 showed that invasion of goat uterine tissue by trophoblast from goat × sheep hybrid fetuses appeared to be more active than normal may be pertinent. In man Dr. W. R. Jones has carried out analyses of maternal ABO blood groups and placental weight(s) from 3688 consecutive confinements, recognizing that the presence of these antigens on the trophoblast was in doubt (see Chapter 6) and that there must have been many other histocompatibility differences between fetus and mother. Since blood group data were not available for the children, the expected proportions of ABO incompatible pregnancies for the O, A, B, and AB maternal groups were estimated from the gene frequencies in the population. The results obtained suggested that disparity between fetus and mother with respect to these antigens was associated with a relatively smaller placenta and vice versa; i.e., the situation appeared to be exactly the opposite of that in mice.

A recent report by Drs. Jenkins and Good, on the other hand, relates placental weight in the human to histocompatibility antigen-dependent reactivity between the maternal and fetal cells. They suggest that histoincompatibility does influence placental weights in humans and that greater disparity is associated with larger placentas.

3. Finally, is the immunity involved a humoral or cellular one? The following experiments relate to this last question.

In the rat, the principles discussed above have been shown to apply (see Fig. 2-7). (a) Fischer females mated with Ag-B locus incompatible DA males produced larger feto-placental units than if mated with males of their own strain; (b) Fischer females presensitized to DA strain tissue antigens and subsequently mated to DA males produced heavier (Fischer × DA)F_1 hybrid feto-placental units than did normal, unsensitized mothers; and (c) the mean weight of (Fischer × DA)F_1 hybrid feto-placental units gestated by Fischer females previously rendered tolerant of the alien DA antigens was significantly less than that of similar progeny borne of normal Fischer mothers. These observations indicate that specific

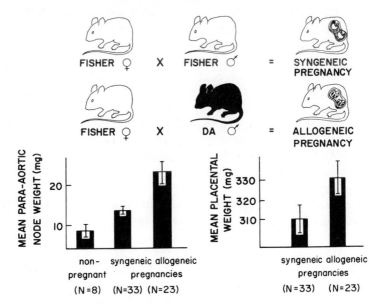

Fig. 2-7. Illustrating the fact that the F_1 hybrid fetuses resulting from matings between Fischer female rats and DA strain males have heavier or larger placentas than syngeneic Fischer fetuses. Comparison of the weights of the para-aortic lymph nodes draining the uteri of virgin, female Fischer rats with those of weight- and age-matched Fischer rats bearing Fischer (syngeneic) and (Fischer × DA)F_1 hybrid (allogeneic) fetuses, respectively, of 18 days' gestation, reveals slight stimulation by syngeneic pregnancies, probably due to fetal tissue-specific antigens (possibly associated with the trophoblast) and a much stronger stimulation by genetically alien fetuses due to their tissue alloantigens. This and other evidence implicates maternal reactivity against the tissue alloantigens of the conceptus as a determinant of the growth rate of the feto-placental unit.

immunologic reactivity on the part of the mother toward the alien cellular antigens of the fertilized eggs that confront her endometrium plays a role, albeit a minor one, in determining the weights of the feto-placental units. If the immunologic reactivity potential of the mother is frustrated by rendering her immunologically tolerant of the tissue antigens of her fetuses, the growth potential of the feto-placental unit will not be fully realized.

If the maternal reactivity against fetal tissue histocompatibility antigens in part determines the weight of the feto-placental units, then the draining para-aortic nodes and/or the spleen, either singly or together, might be the most likely generators of the pertinent effector cellular or humoral immunological responses contributing to this phenomenon. To elucidate the influence of these two lymphoid organs on the feto-placental weights, panels of Fischer females had either their bilateral para-aortic nodes or their spleens removed prior to mating with DA strain males. Both procedures significantly reduced the mean weights of the feto-placental units when these were compared with those of animals in control and sham operated series.

Since the spleen is the principal seat of the synthesis of antibodies when antigenic material is presented via the intravenous route, it seemed likely that humoral antibodies might be the principal mediators of placental and fetal growth in utero. To test this premise, panels of Fischer females mated with DA males were passively immunized with Fischer Anti-DA tissue hyperimmune serum every third day, starting after implantation, and continuing until the end of the gestation period. It was found that the feto-placental units of these females were significantly heavier than those of the allogeneic control group and heavier than those of females given normal Fischer serum throughout gestation.

The results discussed in this chapter give us good grounds for the belief that immunogenetic differences between the fetus and its mother, and the immunologic status of the mother with regard to the histocompatibility antigens of the fetus, exert some influence on the behavior of the trophoblast as it invades the maternal uterine tissue in the process of the formation of the placenta. The greater the genetic disparity involved, the larger or heavier will be the feto-placental unit. These parameters can be augmented by prior local or systemic immunization of the mother against the antigens concerned or minimized by interfering with her capacity to respond. The exact factors that limit the normal, quasi-malignant invasion of the maternal uterine tissue by the trophoblast have yet to be elucidated. The fact that limitation occurs when females are mated to genetically similar males, where there are no histocompatibility differences, rules out the possibility that the transplantation immunity system plays the only part in this important immunologic coexistence. There is certainly the possibility that developmental antigens of some kind also play a part.

REFERENCES

Barker, C. F., and Billingham, R. E. 1968. "The role of afferent lymphatics in the rejection of skin homografts." *J. Exp. Med.* **128**:197–221.

Barker, C. F., and Billingham, R. E. 1973. "Immunologically privileged sites and tissues." Ciba Foundation Symposium 15. *Corneal Graft Failure.* Elsevier-Excerpta Medica. North-Holland. pp. 79–99.

Beer, A. E., and Billingham, R. E. 1970. "Implantation, transplantation, and epithelial-mesenchymal relationships in the rat uterus." *J. Exp. Med.* **132**:721–736.

Beer, A. E., and Billingham, R. E. 1974. "Host response to intra-uterine tissue, cellular and fetal allografts." *J. Reprod. Fertil., Suppl.* **21**:59–88.

Billingham, R. E. 1968. "The biology of graft-versus-host reactions." In *Harvey Lectures,* Series 62. Academic Press, New York. pp. 21–78.

Billington, W. D. 1964. "Influence of immunological dissimilarity of mother and foetus on size of placenta in mice." *Nature* (London) **202**:317–318.

Billington, W. D. 1965. "The invasiveness of transplanted mouse trophoblast and the influence of immunological factors." *J. Reprod. Fertil.* **10**:343–352.

Billington, W. D. 1970. "Immunology in relation to the placental trophoblast extensions from the placenta." *Proc. Roy. Soc. Med.* **63**:5–14.

Clarke, A. G. 1971. "The effects of maternal pre-immunization on pregnancy in the mouse." *J. Reprod. Fert.* **24**:369–375.

Clarke, B., and Kirby, D. R. S. 1966. "Maintenance of histocompatibility polymorphisms." *Nature* (London) **211**:999–1000.

Finkel, S. I., and Lilly, F. 1971. "Influence of histoincompatibility between mother and foetus on placental size in mice." *Nature* (London) **234**:102–103.

Grebe, S., and Streilein, J. W. 1976. "Graft-versus-host reactions: a review." *Adv. Immunol.* **22**:119.

Hancock, J. L., McGovern, P. T., and Stamp, J. T. 1968. "Failure of gestation of goat-sheep hybrids in goats and sheep." *J. Reprod. Fert., Suppl.* **3**:29–36.

James, D. A. 1965. "Effects of antigenic dissimilarity between mother and foetus on placental size in mice." *Nature* (London) **205**:613–614.

James, D. A. 1967. "Some effects of immunological factors on gestation in mice." *J. Reprod. Fertil.* **14**:265–275.

Jenkins, D. M., and Good, S. 1972. "Mixed lymphocyte reaction and placentation." *Nature* (London) New Biology, **240**:211–212.

Jones, W. R. 1968. "Immunological factors in human placentation." *Nature* (London) **218**:480.

Kirby, D. R. S. 1968. "Transplantation and pregnancy." *In Human Transplantation* (F. T. Rapaport and J. Dausset, ed.). Grune and Stratton, New York and London, pp. 565–586.

Kirby, D. R. S. 1970. "The egg and immunology." *Proc. Roy. Soc. Med.* **63**:59–61.

Mullen, R. J., and Carter, S. C. 1973. "Efficiency of transplanting normal, zona-free, and chimeric embryos to one and both uterine horns of inbred and hybrid mice." *Biol. Reprod.* **9**:111–115.

Schlesinger, M. 1962. "Uterus of rodents as site for manifestation of transplantation immunity against transplantable tumors." *J. Natl. Cancer Inst.* **28**:927–945.

Chapter 3

Autoimmunity and Immunoregulatory Mechanisms

An essential feature of our immunological defense system is its subtle ability to discriminate between "self" and "nonself" material, in addition to its capacity to make the long familiar distinction between different nonself or foreign agents and substances such as microbial pathogens or serum proteins from different species. Inability to discriminate between self and nonself could lead to the synthesis of antibodies and/or effector lymphocytes directed against specific components of the individual's *own* body (autoimmunization), which might have pathologic consequences. Fortunately protective mechanisms exist in the body that normally prevent recognition of self components as antigens by the lymphoid system and if self-components do come to be recognized to minimize the risk of lesions being produced.

So-called autoimmune diseases are those in which an autoantibody or sensitized lymphocytes are present that react with specific host tissues or cells *in vitro* and *in vivo*. It must be emphasized, however, that the association of specific immunologic effector agents with a particular autoimmune disease does not necessarily imply a causal relationship—they may be innocent concomitants.

There are various organ-specific diseases with corresponding organ-specific antibodies affecting the brain, the adrenal gland, the testis, and the skin, of which Hashimoto's disease of the thyroid is a familiar, well-studied example. In this disease specific lesions occur in the thyroid characterized by invasion by mononuclear cells (lymphocytes, macrophages, and plasma cells) from the bloodstream, destruction of follicular cells, and the formation of lymphocytic germinal centers. Associated with these lesions there is production of circulating antibodies specific for certain components of the organ.

Two important mechanisms that are generally believed to play important roles in our protection against the risk of reacting immunologically against self-components are (1) the development of immunologic tolerance of the majority of these and (2) the physiological sequestration of others.

41

IMMUNOLOGIC TOLERANCE AND ITS POSSIBLE ROLE IN DEVELOPMENT

It has been shown experimentally that exposure of very young animals to living allogeneic cells or to a variety of noncellular antigenic materials including heterologous plasma proteins, early in life before their ability to react against these antigens has properly developed may result in a lasting, specific impairment of their ability to react against these antigens later in life—i.e., they have become *tolerant* of the antigens concerned. In 1950 Burnet and Fenner suggested that this mechanism would afford a means whereby individuals become unresponsive to their own body constituents —i.e., they become *self-tolerant*. According to this hypothesis, inoculation of genetically foreign cells or other antigens into very young hosts "tricks them," as Roitt puts it, "into treating these as 'self-components' in later life." It is important to emphasize that ability to become tolerant is not the prerogative of very young animals; animals of *any* age can become tolerant of an antigen. In an operational sense, however, it is usually much more difficult to render immunologically mature subjects tolerant. At whatever age tolerance is induced, persistence of antigenic material seems to be essential to maintain the unresponsive state in being. Moreover, tolerance is not an all or none phenomenon—one can have incomplete tolerance reflected by a demonstrably impaired capacity to react against a particular antigen or complete tolerance in which no reactivity is demonstrable.

Studies on the induction of tolerance to BSA (bovine serum albumin) in adult mice, by Dr. N. A. Mitchison of University College, London, revealed that repeated, very low-dosage inocula of this antigen (in microgram amounts) induced unresponsiveness, whereas intermediate doses (of the order of 100 μg) caused sensitization. Increasing the dosage still further (to about 10,000 μg), however, also resulted in unresponsiveness to subsequent challenge with the antigen. Thus, at least with some antigens, we have so-called "low-zone" and "high-zone" tolerance in terms of the dosage requirements for induction of this type of specific immunologic unresponsiveness.

Although subjected to a great deal of speculation and investigation since it was discovered more than 20 years ago, the phenomenon of immunological tolerance still awaits a fully satisfactory explanation. It is generally believed that administration of antigen under conditions known to cause unresponsinveness results in either the death or the inactivation, rather than the stimulation, of specific clones of antigen-sensitive lymphocytes. This readily accounts for self-tolerance since all lymphocytes having receptors capable of reacting with antigenic determinants associated with self-components would be inactiviated or eliminated, leaving behind in a fully operational state only those lymphocytes with receptors for non-self-determinants to form the basis of the host's potential repertoire of immunologic responses.

Since the phenomenon of tolerance was discovered, the existence of two different classes of antigen-sensitive cells has been established—*T lymphocytes* (which are thymus-dependent and responsible for cellular immunity) and *B lymphocytes* (which are bursa-, or bursa-equivalent-dependent). When stimulated by antigen these B cells develop into plasma cells that are responsible for the synthesis of circulating antibody. The ability of B cells to react against certain antigens (so-called thymus-dependent antigens) requires cooperation with T cells. Possibly, as Mitchison has suggested, T lymphocytes serve as "helpers" that pick up an antigen via one of its many different determinants and present other determinants to B lymphocytes. By presenting antigen to B cells in this way, the helper cells may constitute a sort of "antigen-focusing" or concentrating mechanism. In some immunologic reactions macrophages may also enter the picture, playing a nonspecific role. Possibly they trap antigen onto their surfaces to which both B and T cells attach by means of their receptor sites. Their close proximity may also facilitate an important interaction between these cells.

It has been established that tolerance can be induced in both B and T lymphocyte populations, though for some antigens there is considerable disparity in the ease with which this is accomplished. B lymphocytes, which have many more receptors on their surfaces than T lymphocytes, seem to require exposure to much higher concentrations of antigen and for longer periods than T lymphocytes to render them unresponsive. Moreover, unresponsiveness seems to persist longer in T cell populations than in B cell populations. For immunologic responses that require the cooperative activity of both T and B cells, however, the induction of, or persistence of, tolerance in one lymphocyte population only, will still be reflected in unresponsiveness on the part of the individual.

SEQUESTERED ANTIGENS

The second mechanism that is believed to help protect individuals from reacting against certain "self-components" is the development and retention of the latter in a physiologically isolated or quarantined environment so that antigen-sensitive cells are denied the exposure to them. As already mentioned, such exposure would normally induce self-tolerance during development or evoke sensitization in later life. Examples are specific proteins present in the lens of the eye and thyroglobulin within the thyroid gland; casein and other proteins secreted in milk; and, as we shall see later, specific components of testis. Thus if the quarantining boundaries of such organs are compromised in adult life by trauma or infection, normally sequestered antigen of which the subject is not tolerant may gain access to the lymphocytes, via draining lymphatic and blood vessels, and autoantibodies and/or effector lymphocytes may be produced.

It is important to realize, however, that the formation of an autoantibody is not necessarily prejudicial to the well-being of the subject. As individuals get older, some of the homeostatic mechanisms that prevent the recognition and treatment of self-components as foreign and antigenic may fail. It has been suggested that some of the resulting autoantibodies may actually help in the disposal of the products of every day "wear and tear" at the cellular and tissue levels. The antibodies that appear after myocardial infarction, presumably in response to the release of normally sequestered antigens in cardiac muscle, appear to be totally harmless.

For most potentially autoantigenic, sequestered body constituents it has been found in experimental animals that injection of simple unmodified saline extracts or homogenates of tissues that are affected by specific autoimmune diseases in man usually fails to elicit antibody formation or the development of lesions. Careful investigation of the thyroid autoantigen, thyroglobulin, by Dr. Ivan Roitt and his associates of the Middlesex Hospital Medical School, London, has revealed that, contrary to previous belief, this substance is not completely sequestered within the follicles of the normal gland. It normally leaks into the extracellular, perifollicular fluid whence it passes via the lymphatics into the bloodstream though in very small amounts. These low concentrations may suffice to induce low-zone tolerance in the T lymphocytes but not in the B lymphocytes. Because of this tolerance to thyroglobulin the T cells may be unable to activate the nontolerant B cells. This situation may apply to other sequestered body constituents.

Ways in which this kind of situation could be compromised to the detriment of the individual include the following: (1) by presentation of the potential autoantigenic determinants on a new or modified carrier protein or other relatively large molecule, as a consequence of some kind of enzyme or pathogen-induced modification; (2) by alteration of the physical mode of presentation of the self-components in some way. It has long been known that when animals are injected with relatively simple saline extracts of certain organs emulsified in mineral oil containing killed tubercle bacilli (Freund's complete adjuvant—hereafter CFA) autoantibodies appear in the serum and destructive inflammatory lesions develop in the organ concerned. For example, as Rose and Witebsky have demonstrated, if rabbits are injected with rabbit thyroglobulin in CFA, they develop anti-thyroglobulin antibodies and thyroiditis that leads to destruction of the architecture of the gland. Microscopically the lesions characterizing this experimentally induced autoimmune disease closely resemble those of human autoimmune thyroiditis as exemplified by Hashimoto's disease.

By essentially similar maneuvers, lesions can be caused to develop in the brain (encephalomyelitis with associated paralysis) by injection of central nervous system tissue; in the adrenal gland, and, as we shall see, in the testis. In the case of the kidney, injection of heterologous glomeruli will stimulate the production of antibodies directed against glomerular basement membranes. These antibodies localize in the recipient's kidneys causing severe glomerulonephritis.

Most of these experimentally procurable autoimmune diseases are consistently transmissible from immunized animals to normal syngeneic hosts by means of viable lymphoid cells and a few are sometimes transmissible by means of immune serum. On the basis of this and other evidence it is believed that the lesions observed are mediated by effector lymphocytes rather than by antibodies, though cooperativity or synergism between these two classes of immunologic effectors cannot be excluded. The close similarity that some of these experimental autoallergies bear to human, organ-specific diseases strengthens the belief that the pathogenesis of the latter is indeed immunologically mediated.

IMMUNOREGULATION BY ANTIBODY

When an animal is exposed to antigenic material, specific antibodies belonging to various immunoglobulin classes appear in a sequential order and the binding affinity of these antibodies for the antigen tends to increase with time. Analysis of these events has indicated that the immune response is subject to the control of regulatory mechanisms. For example, the physical and biological properties of the antigen determines the specificity and other characteristics of the antibodies produced; in addition, the dosage and route of administration of the antigen determine whether its influence will be predominantly immunogenic or tolerogenic. The various immunoglobulins themselves also appear to exert an important regulatory influence on their *own* synthesis that has been subjected to intensive investigation and will only be dealt with briefly here.

The classic observation indicating that antibodies can suppress their own synthesis was the finding that injection of a mixture of specific antibody and toxin abolished the toxic effects of the latter as well as its ability to elicit a detectable immune response. The treated subject was primed, however, in the sense that he responded to subsequent injection of toxin or the corresponding natural infection by a normal secondary response.

Antibody suppression of the immune response is highly specific, which has lent support to the belief that the suppression must turn upon combination of antibody with specific antigen; and antibodies suppress the primary response more readily than they do the secondary immune response. Two additional examples of immunosuppression by antibody are (1) the prevention of Rh isoimmunization by the administration of anti-Rh antibodies shortly after the delivery of an Rh-positive baby by an Rh-negative woman (see Chapter 11) and (2) immunologic enhancement.

Immunologic enhancement may be defined as the prolongation of survival of allografts of tumors or of certain normal tissues or organs obtained by treating the hosts with isoantibodies directed against the transplantation antigens of the alien cells. This phenomenon is paradoxical in the sense that the antibody fails to curtail graft survival (or tumor growth) as might have been expected but actually interferes with the development or effectuation of the normal immunological rejection process. Transplantation systems are complicated from the immunologic viewpoint. The antigens are associated with cells that are usually capable of replicating and, depending on their "tissue type," these display quantitative variation in their expression of the determinants corresponding to histocompatibility alleles at a multiplicity of histocompatibility loci. Cells vary in their sensitivity to complement-dependent cytotoxic antibodies *in vitro* and *in vivo*. There is no doubt, however, that enhancement does reflect an antibody-mediated suppression of the immune response, essentially similar to that obtainable with much simpler, nonreproducing antigens. In support of this thesis is evidence that isoantibody-treated recipients of allogenic tumor cells fail to develop a normal humoral or cell-mediated immune response. Especially important is the latter shortcoming since, although allografts elicit a dual modality of immunologic response, mediated by lymphocytes and humoral antibodies, respectively, for nearly all types of solid tissue allograft, it is the *cellular* component that is responsible for their destruction. It is important to note that the enhancement phenomenon is not demonstrable in those circumstances in which the "target" allograft cells employed are susceptible to the cytotoxic action of humoral antibodies and complement, as in the case of many leukemias, and normal hematopoietic and lymphoid cells. If appropriate steps are taken to remove or diminish the effect of these cytotoxic antibodies, however, cells of these types are amenable to enhancement. For example, leukemias can be made susceptible to the induction of enhancement by removal of the Fc (complement fixing) fragment of the antibodies.

MECHANISM OF IMMUNOSUPPRESSION BY ANTIBODY

Antibody may exert its immunosuppressive effect at one or other, or both, of two different levels: peripherally or centrally. Peripheral inhibition implies action of antibody on potentially immunogenic sites of the antigen. In the case of enhancement, there is also an efferent protection of antibody-coated cells against destruction by sensitized "killer" lymphocytes.

A central mechanism of immunosuppression implies an effect on antibody-forming cells or their precursors, or the precursors of cellular immunity. Here there are grounds for belief that the suppression is mediated by immune complexes—mixtures of antibody and antigen—acting on the surface of the cells. Experiments by Drs. Diener and Feldman, at the Hall Institute in Melbourne, Australia, using the H antigen of *Salmonella adelaide,* have shown that immunologic tolerance is inducible both *in vivo* and *in vitro* by very small amounts of antigen in the presence of specific antibody. These workers postulated that the central immunosuppressive effect of immune complexes is due to the formation of a lattice of immune complexes on the antigen receptors of lymphocytes. This would lead to interlinkage between the receptors that might induce tolerance. However the possibility of a direct, immune complex-induced lytic effect on the lymphocytes was not excluded.

Since there is now evidence that transferred antibodies can protect transplanted organ allografts—especially renal allografts in rats—against immune destruction, there are now grounds for optimism that the principle of antibody suppression may be applicable to organ allotransplantation in man. It may also be applicable to the treatment of autoimmune diseases: Appropriate noncytotoxic antibodies, by combining with target tissues, may be capable of protecting them from destruction by sensitized lymphocytes.

Apart from passive enhancement by transfer of isoantibody, animals can be actively enhanced in respect of subsequent tissue allografts through active immunization with homogenates, desiccates, and other nonliving preparations from the donor strain. This affords a possible explanation for the existence of autoantibodies in the serum of individuals that display no lesions in the corresponding organ. Leakage of organ-specific antigenic material may have elicited the formation of protective or "blocking" antibodies capable of impairing the development of a cellular immune response and/or the ability of effector lymphocytes to interact with the target tissue or cells.

SUPRESSOR T CELLS AND THEIR ROLE IN IMMUNOREGULATION

Although the findings of numerous investigators over the past decade have highlighted the role that antibody plays in enhancement of tumor growth, maintenance of some forms of immunologic unresponsiveness or paralysis, and prolongation of the survival of tissue and organ allografts, its mechanisms of action remain somewhat equivocal. Recent work has revealed the existence of a category of lymphocytic cells that can exert an active suppressive influence on immune responses. These are known as suppressor T cells because of their function and probable thymic derivation. They can inhibit antibody synthesis by B lymphocytes, exert a suppressive or restraining influence on graft-versus-host reactions, block Mixed Leukocyte Culture Reactions, inhibit tumor cell proliferation, and establish tolerance or unresponsiveness to certain antigens when adoptively transferred to a naive host.

The immunoregulatory influence of these suppressor T cells has been established in a variety of experimental systems in many different laboratories. Dr. Richard Gershon and his associates at Yale University School of Medicine were unable to induce tolerance of sheep erythrocytes (SRBC's) in mice that had been treated in such a way as to deplete their T cells. However, restitution of the tolerance—responsiveness of these animals to this antigen could be accomplished by replacement of their T cells. Furthermore, when T cells from normal, nontolerant mice were transferred to animals tolerant of SRBC's, they failed to make antibody in their new hosts. These workers also found that if spleen cells were transferred from mice that were tolerant of SRBC to normal mice, the latter also behaved as if they were tolerant. Treatment of spleen cells from tolerant donors with anti-theta serum (which reacts with determinants on T cells), however, abolished their ability to transfer tolerance. These observations suggest that certain populations of T cells are needed to suppress the immune response in animals rendered tolerant by exposure to antigen and that, once a state of tolerance has been induced, suppressor T cells prevent nontolerant lymphoid cells in the animal from responding to the antigen.

Dr. Philip Baker and co-workers at the National Institute of Allergy and Infectious Diseases immunized mice with type III pneumococcal polysaccharide and found that treating them with antilymphocyte serum (ALS) increased their response to this antigen. Infusion of thymocytes from normal, syngeneic donors into experimental subjects abrogated this increased response. These investigators also found that *nude* mice, which are congenitally athymic and lack T lymphocytes, responded better against this antigen than did normal, euthymic mice, but treatment of sensitized nude mice with ALS did not further increase their response. They concluded that normal mice have "amplifier cells" that, in the absence of an adequate number of suppressor T cells, increase the animal's response to the antigen in question. Since the nude mouse lacks both of these cell types, treatment with ALS doesn't increase their response.

When female BALB/c mice, whose immunoglobulin has one antigenic genetic marker or allotypic specificity, are mated with males of the SJL/L strain, whose immunoglobulin has a different allotypic specificity, the F_1 hybrid progeny will have both immunoglobulin allotypes. If the BALB/c females have been immunized with the paternal strain immunoglobulin before mating, however, there is marked, long-lasting suppression of the paternal allotype in the majority of the F_1 progeny—the phenomenon of *allotype suppression* (see page 159). The Herzenbergs, of Stanford University School of Medicine, have shown that a class of T lymphocytes is responsible for this phenomenon. When irradiated BALB/c mice were reconstituted with splenic cells from normal hybrid progeny, they began to produce immunoglobulin of both parental allotypes. When mixtures of equal numbers of spleen cells from normal and suppressed hybrid donors were injected into irradiated BALB/c mice, however, much less of the paternal immunoglobulin allotype was produced. If spleen cells from the suppressed F_1 donors were treated with anti-theta antibody before mixing with spleen cells from normal hybrids, and then transferred to irradiated BALB/c hosts, both immunoglobulin allotypes were produced in comparable amounts.

On the basis of their finding that spleens from older animals contain far fewer suppressor T cells than spleens from younger animals, Dr. Hugh Folch and colleagues from Yale have suggested that a decrease in suppressor T cells with age may account for the reported increase in incidence of autoantibodies with advancing age. They and many other workers are developing the concept that suppressor T cell activity is essential for the control of the normal immune response and that malfunction of this control system could lead to the production of aberrant or excess antibodies or even of antibodies capable of attacking the individual's *own* tissues, i.e., autoimmunity.

Direct supportive evidence for this concept has been forthcoming. For example, Alfred Steinberg and co-investigators have demonstrated that NZB strain mice, which normally develop an autoimmune disease closely resembling systemic lupus erythematosis in man, suffer a precocious loss of suppressor T cells from their lymphomyeloid complex before the development of autoimmune disease.

There is also suggestive evidence that having too many suppressor T cells may be harmful and lead to an immunologic dysfunction such as hyporeactivity to the antigens of chemically induced tumors.

Recent work from several laboratories would suggest that suppressor T cells secrete substances that turn other cells on or off and that this action requires protein synthesis but not cell division on the part of the T cell.

The immunoregulatory mechanism operational during allogeneic pregnancy that allows the successful survival of the feto-placental allograft

50   AUTOIMMUNITY AND IMMUNOREGULATORY MECHANISMS

remains somewhat enigmatic even at the present time. The immune system of the pregnant host and its plethora of responses is highly complex. As attempts are made to synthesize the role of suppressor T cells and other factors on a backdrop of what is already known about antibody-mediated immunoregulation, the mysteries of immunologic coexistence in pregnancy may aggregate into a coherent picture.

REFERENCES

Allison, A. C., Denman, A. M., and Barnes, R. D. 1971. "Cooperating and controlling functions of thymus derived lymphocytes in relation to autoimmunity." *Lancet* **II**:135–140.

Baker, P., Stashak, P., Amsbaugh, D., Prescott, B. 1974. "Regulation of the antibody response to type III pneumococcal polysaccharide: II. Mode of action of thymic-derived suppressor cells." *J. Immunol.* **112**:404–409.

Barthold, D., Kysela, S., and Steinberg, A. 1974. "Decline in suppressor T cell function with age in female NZB mice." *J. Immunol.* **112**:9–16.

Benjamin, D. C. 1975. "Evidence for specific suppression in the maintenance of immunologic tolerance." *J. Exp. Med.* **141**:635–645.

Billingham, R. E. 1974. "Immunological tolerance and its possible role in development." In *Concepts of development* (J. Lash and J. R. Whittaker, ed.). Sinauer Associates, Inc., Stanford, Conn., pp. 272–292.

Brent, L. 1975. "Introduction to the symposium on tolerance and enhancement." In *Transplantation Today,* Vol. 3 (M. Schlesinger, R. E. Billingham, and F. T. Rapaport, ed.). Grune and Stratton, Inc., New York, pp. 337–343.

Burnet, F. M. 1972. *Auto-immunity and auto-immune disease.* F. A. Davis, Philadelphia.

Diener, E., and Feldman, M. 1970. "Antibody-mediated suppression of the immune response *in vitro*. II. A new approach to the phenomenon of immunological tolerance." *J. Exp. Med.* **132**:31–43.

French, M. E., and Batchelor, J. R. 1972. "Enhancement of renal allografts in rats and man." *Transpl. Rev.* **13**:115–141.

Gershon, R. K. 1974. "T cell control of antibody production." In *Contemporary Topics in Immunology* (M. D. Cooper and N. L. Warner, ed.). Plenum Press, New York, pp. 1–39.

Gershon, R., Mokyr, M., Mitchell, M. 1974. "Activation of suppressor T cells by tumor cells and specific antibody." *Nature* **250**:594–596.

Herzenberg, L. A., Chan, E. L., Ravitch, M. M., Riblet, R. J., and Herzenberg, L. A. 1973. "Active suppression of immunoglobulin allotype synthesis. III. Identification of T cells as responsible for suppression by cells from spleen, thymus, lymph node and bone marrow." *J. Exp. Med.* **137**:1311–1324.

Hildemann, W. H., and Mullen, Y. 1973. "The weaker the histoincompatibility, the greater the effectiveness of specific immunoblocking antibodies: A new immunogenetic rule of transplantation." *Transpl. Proc.* **5**:617–620.

Kirchner, H., Muchmore, A. V., Chused, T. M., Holden, H. T., and Herberman, R. B. 1975. "Inhibition of proliferation of lymphoma cells and T lymphocytes by suppressor cells from spleens of tumor-bearing mice." *J. Immunol.* **114**:206–210.

Mitchison, N. A. 1971. "Suppression of immune responses by antigen." In *Immunological diseases* (M. Samter, ed.). Little, Brown and Co., Boston, pp. 148–160.

Möller, G., and Britton, S. 1971. "Regulation of the immune response by antibody." In *Immunological diseases* (M. Samter, ed.). Little, Brown and Co., Boston, pp. 136–147.

Nisbet, N. W., and Elves, M. W., ed. 1971. "Immunological tolerance to tissue antigens." Orthopaedic Hospital, Oswestry, England.

Roitt, I. M. 1971. *Essential immunology.* Blackwell, Oxford.

Rose, N. R., and Witebsky, E. 1971. "Experimental thyroiditis." In *Immunological diseases* (M. Samter, ed.). Little, Brown and Co., Boston, pp. 1179–1197.

Schwartz, R. S. 1971. "Immunoregulation by antibody." In *Progress in immunology* (D. B. Amos, ed.). First International Congress of Immunology, Academic Press, New York, pp. 1081–1091.

Snell, G. D. 1970. "Immunologic enhancement." *Surg., Gynecol., Obstet.* **130**:1109–1119.

Weigle, W. O. 1971. "Immunologic unresponsiveness." In *Immunobiology* (R. A. Good and D. W. Fisher, ed.). Sinauer Associates, Inc., Stanford, Conn., pp. 123–134.

Chapter 4

Antigens of the Male Reproductive System

The various components of the male reproductive system, which include the testis, the epididymis, the vas deferens and its ampulla, the seminal vesicle, coagulating gland, bulbourethral (Cowper's) gland and the prostate (see Fig. 4-1), do not attain functional maturation until relatively late in development. Moreover, some of their secretory products (so far as these have been defined) are unique and are normally discharged *outside* the body in the ejaculate. There is thus a strong *prima facie* case that here we may be dealing with highly specialized cellular and other components that have differentiated, or been synthesized, in sequestered sites and of which the subject has not had the opportunity to become tolerant during his development and to which his immunologic response machinery is not normally exposed during later life.

EARLY STUDIES

Interest in the distinctive immunological properties of the components of male ejaculates and of the organs that produce them stems from the independent discovery by Carl Landsteiner in 1899 and by Elie Metchnikoff and S. Metalnikoff in 1900 that the serum of guinea pigs injected with semen or homogenized testes from men, bulls, rabbits, or other guinea pigs acquires the capacity to agglutinate and immobilize living spermatozoa of these various species *in vitro*. Considerable cross-reactivity was observed between the spermatozoa of closely related species. In 1909 Adler made the important additional observation that guinea pigs produced autoantibodies following injection of their *own* spermatozoa. Brain was the only other tissue with whose antigens these antitestis or antispermatozoal antibodies would react. By 1961, according to the late Dr. Albert Tyler of the California Institute of Technology, the results of more than 150 independent experiments had been published in which guinea pigs, rabbits, rats, women, and other subjects had been immunized with seminal materials from their own or from different species, principally to study

52

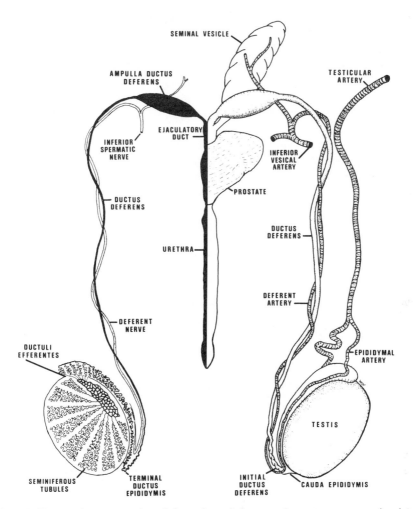

Fig. 4-1. Diagramatic representation of the male genital system. Spermatozoa are produced in enormous numbers by the proliferation and specialization of cells in the germinal epithelium lining the seminiferous tubules of the testis. From these seminiferous tubules, the spermatozoa pass via a plexiform system of epithelialized channels known as the rete testis to the ductuli efferentes. The latter discharge into the single, very long but highly convoluted ductus epididymis that terminates in the ductus or vas deferens, the excretory duct of the testis. The ductus deferens dilates into an ampulla near to the distal end of which it is joined by the duct of a large gland, the seminal vesicle. Finally, as a short, straight ejaculatory duct, the ductus deferens passes through the body of the large prostate gland and opens into the urethra. The numerous excretory ducts of the prostate gland open directly into the urethra. During ejaculation, as a consequence of the contraction of smooth muscle, spermatozoa that are stored in the epididymis are rapidly transported along the ductus deferens and discharged into the urethra. In addition to spermatozoa, semen includes special secretions from the epididymis, the seminal vesicles, the prostate, and glands of Cowper and of Littré. These secretions are important for the maintenance of the spermatozoa and for enabling fertilization to take place. (From W. B. Neaves. "Biological aspects of vasectomy." In *Handbook of Physiology, Male Reproductive System,* edited by Roy O. Greep and D. W. Hamilton. Washington, D.C.: Am. Physiol. Soc., 1975, Sec. 7, Vol. V, Chap. 18, pp. 383–404.)

their antifertility effect. Tyler's careful survey of this work led him to conclude that no reliable means had been discovered for the immunological control of fertility in any species, despite the fact that many of these experiments had resulted in the production of antibodies that, if added to spermatozoa *in vitro,* destroyed their capacity to fertilize.

Work in this important field was greatly facilitated by the discovery in the early 1950's by Dr. Guy Voisin and his associates in Paris and by Dr. Jules Freund and co-workers in the United States that in the guinea pig spermatogenesis can be suppressed following the injection of homogenates of allogeneic or autologous testis, suspensions of spermatozoa, or extracts of these materials. Their incorporation into an adjuvant, CFA, was found to be necessary to obtain consistently reproducible results.

Manifestations of the Allergic Response to Testicular Antigen

The allergic response to testicular antigen develops within about 2-8 weeks of a single injection of the material in adjuvant. It is characterized by congestion and serous edema in most of the intertubular tissue spaces of the testis and there are foci of perivascular cellular infiltration—by macrophages, plasma cells, and lymphocytes. Compared with the dramatic breakdown of the germinative epithelium in the seminiferous tubules, however, the vascular and inflammatory changes in the interstitial connective tissue are relatively trivial. Vacuolation of germinal cells is first observed in the spermatids and spermatocytes and finally affects the spermatogonia. This is followed by exfoliation so that within 8 weeks the tetes are devoid of spermatogenic tissue except for spermatogonia and Sertoli cells. Androgen production by the Leydig cells of the interstitial tissue continues, however, and neither these cells nor any other connective tissue elements reflect any adverse influences. The accessory organs of reproduction remain perfectly normal in appearance.

The azoospermia resulting from germinal cell destruction renders the animal sterile for several months. Although this experimentally induced sterility is spontaneously reversible through the reappearance of normal spermatozoa in the ejaculates within 6–8 months, periodic reimmunization will prevent repopulation of the seminiferous tubules and so maintain sterility.

Concomitant with the appearance of the testicular lesions, antispermatozoal antibodies appear in the bloodstream. These are of low titer and can be detected by a variety of techniques including systemic anaphylaxis, skin reactions of the immediate type, passive cutaneous anaphylaxis (PCA), Schultze-Dale reactions, complement fixation, cytotoxicity, fluorescent staining following uptake by normal testical tissue, hemagglutination, and precipitin reactions. The immune sera also display agglutinating and cytotoxic activity toward spermatozoa *in vivo* and have a lytic effect on the acrosomes of spermatozoa and spermatids. The animals also develop the ability to give cutaneous reactions of the delayed type following challenge with testicular or spermatozoal extracts. Even if the sensitizing antigen is not incorporated in CFA, repeated inoculation of guinea pigs with adult testicular extract over a several-month period may also elicit testicular damage.

Other species in which testicular lesions have been produced by experimental autoimmunization include mice, rats, rabbits, rhesus monkeys, bulls, and man (in which volunteer prostatic carcinoma patients were used). The guinea pig, however, is certainly the most susceptible species. It is interesting to note in the rabbit that aspermatogenesis and epididymitis can be induced in a normal testis by local, intense freezing of the contralateral organ—i.e., by cryoautoimmunization, in the absence of an adjuvant.

Location and Nature of the Antigenic Stimulus Associated with Testis

Observations that (1) spermatozoa, as antigen, will induce the development of testicular lesions; (2) testicular homogenates from newborn guinea pigs (but not from 14-day-old guinea pigs) or from mature guinea pigs rendered azoospermic by prior sensitization fail to induce testicular lesions; and (3) fluorescent microscopy indicates localization of antitesticular antibodies in the cytoplasm of the spermatids and the acrosomes of spermatozoa suggest that the autoantigenic moiety of the testis is associated principally if not exclusively with the later cell stages of spermatogenesis.

Antigenic material has been extracted from testis and purified to the point where as little as 4 μg of material incorporated in CFA will induce aspermatogenesis in the guinea pig. Active preparations are highly thermostable and contain a significant proportion of glycoprotein material, though the degree of molecular purity of these preparations remains unknown.

Immunopathogenesis of the Lesions in Experimental Allergic Orchitis

Most authorities believe that lymphocytes are the principal if not the exclusive immunologic effectors responsible for the lesions of experimental allergic orchitis on the basis of the following findings: (1) The use of CFA is usually essential to procure the lesions. (2) The severity of the lesions correlates better with the intensity of the delayed skin reactions given by an animal than with the titers of its circulating antibodies. (3) Transfer of viable lymph node cells from sensitized animals to normal, syngeneic hosts confers the ability to give delayed skin reactions as well as inciting testicular lesions. (4) Transfer of putatively immune serum from sensitized donors fails to induce aspermatogenesis or cause testicular lesions and even direct intratesticular inoculation of antibody is nonpathogenic. (5) Finally, passively transferred labeled antibodies do not localize in the seminiferous tubules.

Close scrutiny of the available data reveals, however, that the case in favor of lymphocytes as the *exclusive* mediators of the testicular lesions is not without its shortcomings. Among these is Voisin and Toulet's important observation that, in male guinea pigs immunized with extracted auto-antigenic material and showing aspermatogenesis, 9% displayed a cutaneous hypersensitivity response alone, 67% had both delayed cutaneous hypersensitivity and humoral antibodies, and 26% had only responded to the antigen by antibody production.

Obviously, to evaluate the possible pathogenic significance of antibody it is necessary to have some idea of the facility with which immunoglobulins can normally gain access to the fluid in the seminiferous tubules or the rete testis. Drs. M. H. Johnson and B. P. Setchel of Cambridge University ingeniously took advantage of the fact that in the ram the secretions of the seminiferous tubules can be collected from the rete testis by means of a cannula inserted via the vasa efferentia. Comparison of the immunoglobulin concentrations in the serum with those in the seminiferous tubule secretions indicated that very little immunoglobulin enters the latter, its concentration being only about 0.2% of that in the serum, though it did have antibody activity. In the ram's seminal plasma the immunoglobulin content is higher, being about 2% of that in the serum. On the basis of these important observations these workers postulated the existence of a highly efficient *blood-testis* barrier that prevents the passage of appreciable amounts of serum proteins, to which the vasculature is highly permeable, from entering the seminiferous tubules from the interstitial tissue. This barrier may therefore be able to prevent the ingress of immunologically significant concentrations of complement-fixing IgG antibody, which is cytotoxic to spermatozoa *in vitro* and which is normally present in low titers in the sera of untreated members of several species, as well as potentially harmful antibodies resulting from immunization with testis. They further suggest that this barrier may also play an important role in preventing the leakage of spermatozoal antigen into the circulation and its engagement with lymphocytes in a manner that might lead to autoimmunization.

Dr. Don Fawcett and co-workers at Harvard University have shown that the blood-testis barrier consists of a system of tight junctional complexes between adjacent Sertoli cells. In effect these cells and their tight junctions delimit a basal compartment in the germinal epithelium containing the spermatogonia and an adluminal component that includes spermatocytes and spermatids. Substances reaching the germ cells in the adluminal compartment must pass through the Sertoli cells. The tight junctional complexes, impermeable to cells and macromolecules, protect the seminiferous tubule contents from the mediators of an immune response and also prevent extravasation of spermatozoa into areas where they could come to the attentions of the patrolling, antigen-reactive lymphocytes (see Fig. 4-2).

Recent sequential studies of the histological changes that occur in the testes and epididymides of guinea pigs inoculated with testicular homogenate in CFA have shown that the initial lesions appear in the rete testis and the vasa efferentia. The relative vulnerability of these structures as compared with testicular tissue is ascribed to the inferiority of the blood-testis barrier at this level. The ducts and their surrounding connective tissue are invaded by mononuclear cells, as well as by eosinophils and macrophages, and phagocytosis of spermatozoa occurs. Secondary spread of these early lesions occurs *backward* from the rete testis into the body of the testis. Two possible explanations for this process are (1) the spread into the testis is a result of the adjacent inflammatory reaction increasing tissue permeability that in turn compromises the blood-testis barrier and enables antibodies and lymphocytic effector cells to enter the seminiferous tubules where they can inflict damage upon the spermatogenic cells and (2) antisperm antibodies and/or lymphocytes may enter the inflamed rete testis, progressively spreading back, by reflux, into the seminiferous tubules where they harm the epithelium and, of course, increase the permeability of the tubules to both cells and antibodies.

Johnson maintains that the induction of testicular damage depends on the immune response overcoming or breaking down the normal "quarantining" barrier that protects the seminiferous tubules. This view is in accord with other workers' observation that, in guinea pigs immunized with testis homogenates in CFA, antibody within the seminiferous tubules becomes demonstrable at the same time as delayed hypersensitivity, strongly suggesting that the presence of antibody in the tubules is dependent on the delayed hypersensitivity. Once this barrier has been compromised, release of antigenic material will probably boost the level of the extant immune response. Restoration of the blood-testis barrier and resequestration of the germinal epithelium is probably essential before spermatogenesis is reestablished.

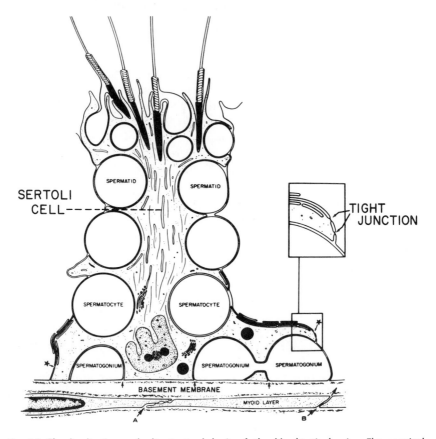

Fig. 4-2. The localization and ultrastructural basis of the blood-testis barrier. The germinal epithelium lining the seminiferous tubules of the testis is composed of cells of two categories: (1) sustentacular or Sertoli cells that are fixed to the basement membrane and extend distally to the lumen, surrounding the spermatogenic cells, and (2) spermatogenic cells of several morphologically distinct types which are successive stages in a continuous process of differentiation of the male germ cells from the earliest precursor spermatogonia which rest on the basement membrane. The spermatogenic cells occupy recesses in the lateral and apical surfaces of the Sertoli cells. The blood-testis barrier is of a dual nature. First, there is a primary barrier made up of a layer of contractile "myoid" cells below the basement membrane that are "sealed" together by occluding junctions (see A). However, the integrity of this barrier is compromised at some sites by the existence of open 200 Å junctions between myoid cells (see B). The second component or tier of the barrier is afforded by adjacent Sertoli cells and the tight junctions that unite their plasma membranes. While substances traversing open junctions in the myoid cell layer do have some portals of direct access to the spermatogonial cells in the basal compartment of the germinal epithelium, to gain access to the spermatocytes and spermatids in the adluminal compartment, they must pass *through* Sertoli cells. (After M. Dym and D. W. Fawcett. "The blood-testis barrier in the rat and the physiologic compartmentation of the seminiferous epithelium." *Biol Reprod.* **3**:308, 1970, Academic Press, Inc., New York.)

Prevention of Experimental
Autoimmune Aspermatogenesis

It is well established that in adult guinea pigs, rabbits, and rats the incidence and severity of experimental allergic encephalomyelitis can be reduced if the subjects are inoculated with homogenates of the corresponding brain tissue in physiological saline either before or after immunization with the same antigen in CFA. As already mentioned (see page 46) this appears to depend on the antibody-mediated suppression of cellular immunity.

Drs. Chutná and Rychlíková, of the Czechoslovak Academy of Sciences, have shown that this principle also applies to experimental autoimmune aspermatogenesis in adult guinea pigs. As we've already seen, immunization of guinea pigs with testicular antigen incorporated in CFA leads to the development of testicular lesions, to delayed cutaneous reactivity, and usually to the synthesis of antibodies that are cytotoxic for spermatozoa in the presence of complement. If the animals are immunized with testicular homogenates, however, in the absence of CFA, testicular lesions, delayed hypersensitivity, and cytotoxic antibodies usually fail to develop, though antibodies demonstrable by immediate cutaneous reactions or by the PCA technique appear. More important, such animals are refractory to subsequent attempts to induce autoimmune aspermatogenesis by reimmunization with testicular antigen in CFA. Furthermore, animals that have received a primary inoculation of the testicular antigen in CFA display suppression of the experimental autoimmune aspermatogenesis if, subsequently, they are repeatedly inoculated with saline homogenates.

Not only do the PCA-type antibodies fail to harm suspensions of testicular cells *in vitro* in the presence of complement, but prior treatment of such cells with this type of antibody will protect them from the otherwise damaging influence of the cytotoxic type of antibody. Presumably competition for antigenic determinant sites on the cell surfaces underlies this phenomenon, which probably also accounts for the *in vivo* findings.

Additional evidence that experimental autoimmune orchitis requires the participation of both a humoral antibody of some kind and delayed hypersensitivity has been presented by Dr. Patricia Brown and her associates of the British Medical Research Council Rheumatism Research Unit. They have shown that guinea pigs injected with a purified testicular extract in incomplete Freund's adjuvant (i.e., which does not contain *Mycobacterium tuberculosis*) fail to develop circulating antibody, delayed hypersensitivity, or testicular lesions. Subsequent injection of these animals with the antigen in complete CFA resulted in the development of delayed hypersensitivity but no testicular lesions or circulating antibody. Repeated inoculation, however, of the recipients of this treatment with serum from guinea pigs immunized with an autoclaved testicular homogenate in CFA caused some of them to develop orchitis.

MUMPS ORCHITIS

Mumps is an acute, communicable virus disease that normally manifests itself by swelling and lesions in the parotid salivary glands that lie just anterior to and beneath the ears. Orchitis is an infrequent manifestation of mumps before puberty but is common in adults, the incidence being about 20%. The symptoms usually develop as the parotitis begins to subside, and in most cases only one testis is affected. Histologically the lesions of mumps orchitis are similar to those of experimental allergic orchitis and a varying degree of atrophy of the affected organ usually results. So far the presence of mumps virus has not been established in the testes of patients with orchitis or in the testes of experimentally affected monkeys. This led to the widely held view that the orchitis results from an autoimmunization, possibly facilitated by initial damage to the blood-testis barrier by the virus. This interpretation is consonant with the observation that mumps orchitis is rare in children before the onset of spermatogenesis. A critical reevaluation of the possibility of cross-reactivity between parotid gland and testis seems worthwhile here. More relevant, perhaps, is evidence of cross-reactivity between the antigens of brain and testis since meningo-encephalitis is a not infrequent complication of mumps. This raises the possibility that the autoimmunity which affects the testis may indeed have been elicited by cross-reacting antigens of the brain.

ANTIGENS OF THE ACCESSORY GLANDS OF REPRODUCTION IN THE MALE

Both human and canine prostatic fluid contains tissue-specific antigens that are absent in other tissues as well as in serum and other secretions of the body. If rabbits are immunized with either homogenates of the prostate or of all the accessory organs incorporated with CFA, antibody reactive with extracts of prostate or each of the other accessory organs develops in high titer. This indicates the sharing of a common antigen by these related tissues and seminal plasma, which is not present elsewhere in the body. Shulman has also produced evidence that, besides this common antigen, rabbit epididymis and seminal plasma share a unique antigen. It is important to note, however, that (with the possible exception of the guinea pig's seminal vesicle, which is very large, and in which both mild and severe lesions have been produced by autoimmunization using CFA) no autoimmune lessions have been produced in any of the accessory organs of reproduction—testis is unique in its susceptibility.

Although rabbits can be made to produce autoantibodies to components of seminal plasma, there is no evidence of naturally occurring autoantibodies to seminal plasma in man.

IMMUNOLOGICAL ASPECTS OF VASECTOMY

Vasectomy, which is being increasingly employed as a means of avoiding pregnancies in humans, was first performed experimentally on dogs by Sir Astley Cooper, a British surgeon, in 1823, and led to the discovery that it did not prevent spermatogenesis and that the epididymis became enlarged to accommodate the sperms. In man, the clinical effects of vas ligation was the subject of much controversy late in the 19th century. Some believed that vasectomy caused no clinical symptoms other than sterility. There were others who believed that it not only caused degeneration of the tubules but hypertrophy of the steroid-secreting cells of the testis leading to sexual rejuvenation. In 1900 a certain Dr. Wood reported that ligation of the vas deferens in patients with prostatic hypertrophy resulted in marked improvement in the majority of patients treated and this mode of therapy was in vogue until the surgical removal of the prostate became more definitive therapy for this troublesome condition of middle-aged males. At this time vasectomy was used to prevent reflux epididymitis that often resulted from surgical prostatectomy. It was not until the early part of the 20th century that vasectomy achieved popularity as a mode of sterilization and was then used mainly for eugenic purposes.

Vasectomy clinics in the United States have mushroomed from a meager 13 in 1970 to nearly 200 by the end of 1972. It is estimated that well over 1 million vasectomies for sterilization were done in 1974. It appears that vasectomy may slightly impair the normal rate of spermatogenesis in man, which is of the order of 50,000 spermatozoa per minute or about 72×10^6 per day. It is pertinent to mention here that in man the total duration of spermatogenesis from the earliest precursor cells, the spermatogonia, and including several mitotic divisions before the two meiotic divisions, to mature spermatozoa, is about 74 days. A normal sperm count is about 60×10^6 per milliliter of seminal plasma.

Since long-term studies on vasectomized animals have revealed that little or no change occurs in the testis itself, it is obvious that the spermatozoa produced must undergo reabsorption somewhere between the testis and the vas deferens. Indeed, even in normal animals, resorption of a high proportion of the spermatozoa produced—of the order of 50%—occurs in the caudal portion of the epididymis. How this occurs awaits elucidation since there is no evidence that epididymal cells are actively phagocytic and normally few macrophages are demonstrable in the lumen of the epididymis. After vasectomy, however, there is a marked increase in the macrophage content of the epididymis, especially in the ductuli efferentes and the caput epididymis and it is generally believed that sperm removal is accomplished by phagocytosis and degradation by these cells.

Long-term studies on vasectomized monkeys, by Dr. Nancy Alexander of the Oregon Regional Primate Research Center, have shown that there is a gradual increase in the level of sperm antibodies in the serum, probably through the mediation of these sperm-removing macrophages. These cells, in addition to fulfilling an antigen-processing role, may also transport antigenic material to seats of immunologic response. Antibody activity may account for the observation that in long-term vasectomized monkeys the spermatozoa present in the ductuli efferentes and the caput epididymis are agglutinated, whereas those in recently vasectomized animals are not. Dr. Alexander has also demonstrated by fluorescent antibody techniques that antigen-antibody complexes with bound complement are laid down in the basal laminas of the efferent ducts, which become thickened, probably as a consequence of an autoantibody reaction to spermatozoal antigens. In the guinea pig this investigator has shown that vasectomy results in a rapid autoimmune disruption of spermatogenesis similar to that observed in male subjects actively immunized with washed isogenic spermatozoa dispensed in complete Freund's adjuvant. This effect was long-lasting and both a cellular and humoral immunity were associated with it.

In man, likewise, there is good evidence from at least five independent investigators that approximately 50% of vasoligated individuals will develop sperm autoantibodies of various types within 1 year of the procedure. The alleged relationship between vasectomy in otherwise healthy young men and the development of a broad variety of unexplained systemic disorders of major magnitude such as thrombophlebitis, prolonged fever, generalized lymphadenopathy, hypergammaglobulinemia, dermatologic conditions, generalized arthritis, interstitial pulmonary fibrosis, glomerulonephritis, hyperinsulinemia, hormonal dysfunction, and a false positive serologic test for syphilis as well as leukemia may appear to challenge the presumed innocuousness of elective vasectomy. Carefully controlled, large-scale studies are necessary, however, to validate these associations.

In men sperm-immobilizing and sperm-agglutinating autoantibodies may also develop in the serum and appear in effective quantities in the ejaculates following inflammatory conditions of the testis or situations leading to occlusion of the vas deferens or the epididymis. Although it is conceivable that the demonstrable autoantibodies to spermatozoa can prejudice fertility, findings to date suggest that autoimmune mechanisms are only responsible for a small proportion of cases of male infertility.

Dr. Ph. Rümke of Amsterdam, in an extensive survey of 2000 infertile males, found that less than 4% had sperm agglutinin titers in their serum and that one-third of these had azoospermia not related to the antibodies but to obstruction of the efferent ducts. This raised the question whether the presence of sperm antibodies in the serum of normospermic males was ever related to infertility. In a 10-year follow-up study of 254 males in this category he found that 36 became fathers. These patients fit into a group with serum or seminal plasma sperm agglutinin titers of 1:32 or less. No pregnancies were engendered by males with titers of 1:512 or over, even if normospermic. Once a serum or seminal plasma sperm agglutinin titer is present, it remains relatively constant over many years and no therapeutic manipulations or agents have been successful in lowering the titer.

In no instances in the human male have sperm agglutinins as such been shown capable of interfering with spermatogenesis.

REFERENCES

Alexander, N. J. 1973. "Autoimmune hypospermatogenesis in vasectomized guinea pigs." *Contraception* **8**:147–164.

Alexander, N. J., Wilson, B. J., and Patterson, G. D. 1974. "Vasectomy: Immunological effects in rhesus monkeys and men." *Fertil. Steril.* **25**:149–156.

Ansbacher, R. 1973. "Vasectomy: Sperm antibodies." *Fertil. Steril.* **24**:788–792.

Brown, P. C., Glynn, L. E., and Holborow, E. J. 1967. "The dual necessity for delayed hypersensitivity and circulating antibody in the pathogenesis of experimental allergic orchitis in guinea pigs." *Immunology* **13**:307–314.

Chutná, J., and Rychlíková, M. 1964. "Prevention and suppression of experimental autoimmune aspermatogenesis in adult guinea pigs." *Folia Biol.* (Praha) **10**:177–186.

Cooper, A. 1845. *Observations on the structure and diseases of the testis.* Lea and Blanchard, Philadelphia.

Fawcett, D. W., Leak, L. V., and Heidger, P. M. 1970. "Electron microscopic observations on the structural components of the blood-testis barrier." *J. Reprod. Fertil. Suppl.* **10**:105–122.

Freund, J., Thompson, G. E., and Lipton, M. M. 1955. "Aspermatogenesis, anaphylaxis and cutaneous sensitization induced in the guinea pig by homologous testicular extract." *J. Exp. Med.* **101**:591–604.

64ANTIGENS OF THE MALE REPRODUCTIVE SYSTEM

Henle, W., Henle, G., and Chambers, L. A. 1938. "Studies on the antigenic structure of some mammalian spermatozoa." *J. Exp. Med.* **68**:335–352.

Howard, P. J., and James, L. P. 1973. "Immunological implications of vasectomy." *J. Urol.* **109**:76–78.

Johnson, M. H. 1970. "Changes in the blood testis barrier of the guinea pig in relation to histological damage following isoimmunization with testis." *J. Reprod. Fertil.* **22**:119–127.

Johnson, M. H., and Setchell, B. P. 1968. "Protein and immunoglobulin content of rete testis fluid of rams." *J. Reprod. Fertil.* **17**:403–406.

Katsh, S., 1969. "Immunological aspects of reproduction." In *Ovum implantation* (M. C. Shelesnyak and G. J. Marcus, ed.). Gordon and Breach, New York, pp. 309–344.

Mancini, R. E., and Andrada, J. A. 1971. "Immunological factors in human male and female infertility." In *Immunological diseases* (M. Samter, ed.). Little, Brown and Company, Boston, pp. 1240–1256.

Neaves, W. B. 1974. "The rat testis after vasectomy: Analysis of the effectiveness of various vasectomy procedures in producing testicular change." *J. Reprod. Fertil.* **40**:39–44.

Roberts, H. J. 1968. "Delayed thrombophlebitis and systemic complications after vasectomy: Possible role of diabetogenic hyperinsulinism." *J. Am. Geriatr. Soc.* **16**:267.

Rümke, Ph., and Hellinga, G. 1959. "Autoantibodies against spermatozoa in sterile men." *Am. J. Clin. Path.* **32**:357–363.

Sackler, A. M., Weltman, A. S., Pandhi, V., and Schwartz, R. 1973. "Gonadal effects of vasectomy and vasoligation." *Science* **179**:293–295.

Shulman, S., Zappi, E., Ahmed, U., and Davis, J. E. 1972. "Immunologic consequences of vasectomy." *Contraception* **5**:269–278.

Toullet, F., Voisin, G. A., and Nemirovsky, M. 1973. "Histoimmunochemical localization of three guinea pig spermatozoal autoantigens." *Immunology* **24**:635–653.

Tyler, A. 1961. "Approaches to the control of fertility based on immunological phenomena." *J. Reprod. Fertil.* **2**:473–506.

Chapter 5

The Antigenic Status of Semen from the Viewpoint of the Female

So far we have been concerned principally with the autoantigenicity of the components of the male reproductive tract and their products—i.e., with the potential reactivity of males to self-components.

Through sexual activity the reproductive tract of the female undergoes repeated inoculation with hundreds of millions of spermatozoa—highly specialized, and usually immunogenetically alien, short-lived cells—together with a minority of other cell types, including leukocytes, suspended in the complex, protein-containing seminal plasma secreted by the specialized accessory reproductive organs of the male. The possible immunological and other effects of this chronic, intermittent process, which is much more frequent in man than in other species, has been subject to repeated investigation as well as to a great deal of speculation. For example, no lesser authority than Charles Darwin, in his *Descent of Man* (1871) made a number of statements relating the profligacy of women to reduced fertility. Despite Carl Hartman's forthright statement that *"much nonsense has been written on this subject"* it is important since, apart from the possibility of explaining some cases of infertility, it also affords one approach to the development of an immunological means of fertility control.

From the female's viewpoint antigenic material or determinants of two classes may be associated with semen. First are *isoantigens* (or alloantigens), such as transplantation or histocompatibility antigens and blood group antigens, which are determined by segregating genes and which can express themselves in both sexes. Whether a female is potentially capable of reacting against the isoantigens present in the semen from a particular male will depend on her own genetic constitution. For example, a woman of blood group A will be incapable of responding immunologically to this antigen if it is present in semen. A given male, of course, will normally be incapable of reacting against his own isoantigens.

Second are *autoantigens,* which are self-components, usually organ- or

65

tissue-specific, against which the individual himself can react. These are constant from one individual to the next throughout the species and consequently individual R can react against D's autoantigens, irrespective of the genetic relationship between them. There is usually considerable cross-reactivity between particular organ-specific antigens of closely related species, a situation that is less common in the case of isoantigens. Although males may have had some "immunologic" experience of seminal autoantigens, this is not the case for females for whom sexual intercourse must necessarily represent their first exposure.

ANTIGENICITY OF SEMEN AND ITS SIGNIFICANCE IN CONTRACEPTION AND INFERTILITY

Dr. Anne McLaren of the University of Edinburgh has shown that after a long course of intraperitoneal injections of syngeneic or allogeneic spermatozoa in the absence of adjuvants, female mice may develop high titers of agglutinins equally effective against spermatozoa from males of *any* murine genotype. Although mating and ovulation occurred normally in such sensitized females, spermatozoa did not appear to reach the site of fertilization in adequate numbers, leading to a lowered rate of fertilization and reduction in litter size. Essentially similar results have been obtained in rabbits, guinea pigs, and cattle by other workers, some of whom have administered the antigenic material in CFA or other adjuvants. In some of her experiments, McLaren included *pertussis* vaccine in her immunization protocol, which increased the serum spermagglutinin titers. Since this did not reduce the fertility of the subjects, it was concluded that the level of sperm antibodies in the blood afforded no meaningful indication of the degree of impairment of their fertility.

Bell and McLaren have reported significant reductions in both litter size and fertilization rate after repeated intraperitoneal injection of female mice with an alum-precipitated supernatant fraction of disrupted spermatozoa. Isolated sperm-head material was ineffective. They noted that whereas freezing the supernatant before injection abolished the capacity of the material to incite sperm agglutinating antibodies, it retained its capacity to impair fertility, indicating that sperm agglutinins were not responsible for the latter. So far no investigator has succeeded in correlating the titer of any kind of antispermatozoal antibody with infertility. Identification of the specific component of spermatozoa that is responsible for prejudicing fertility is clearly an important issue since it may indicate the mechanism of the process. Antigenic determinants associated with the cell surface of the spermatozoa are the *prima facie* candidates, and a complement-dependent cytotoxic antibody is the most likely immunologic effector.

Currently there is tremendous interest in the immunological approach to contraception by "vaccination." Apart from using spermatozoa as antigen, some workers are exploring the use of cross-reacting material such as fetuin, which is present in fetal calf serum. By chemical manipulation it may prove possible to "construct" an immunogen that is more potent than native spermatozoa from the viewpoint of vaccination against conception. As we've already seen, the idea of birth control by immunization of women is by no means new—it was proposed by Meaker in 1922—though there has been no convincing evidence of clinical success to date.

As far as it goes, the evidence from animal experiments is encouraging. One gains the impression, however, that too little of the right kind of antibody gains access to the female reproductive tract. Perhaps topical application of potent antigenic preparations may result in the local formation and secretion across the epithelium of the reproductive tract of effective concentrations of IgA antibody that may form a local defense mechanism against "unwanted" spermatozoa. The problem is analogous to that of devising an effective means of vaccination against respiratory infections.

A factor capable of agglutinating spermatozoa is demonstrable in the serum of both young and adult virgin females of many species and some investigators have regarded this as a naturally occurring sperm autoantibody. Dr. Barry Boettcher and his associates at the University of Newcastle, Australia, have recently presented cogent evidence, however, that indicates that sperm-agglutinating activity in the sera of both pregnant and virgin women may be due to a lipoprotein-steroid conjugate rather than to immunoglobulins.

Under certain conditions, however, spermatozoa or other antigens present in seminal plasma might stimulate antibody production in women and account for some cases of infertility. Recent studies involving over 500 women with primary or secondary infertility showed sperm isoantibodies in 289. Dr. Seymor Katsh has found that antibodies to seminal components are persistently detectable in the serum and cervical mucus of certain patients with idiopathic sterility. However, attempts involving the cooperation of prostitutes and other volunteers to relate antibody response to the degree of coital exposure to seminal material have been unsuccessful or have yielded equivocal results. Recently Dr. Jan Behrman has shown that a significant decrease in antibody titer can be achieved by occlusive (condom) "therapy" and that 50–60% of these hitherto sterile patients will subsequently conceive. The antibodies detectable include complement fixing, agglutinating, immobilizing, or skin sensitizing (PCA—i.e., passive cutaneous anaphylaxis). Various lines of evidence suggest that the infrequently encountered high antibody titers result from normal or pathological conditions that favor the deposition of large numbers of sperms into the uterus where they are rapidly absorbed. Experimentally it has been shown that wounding of the reproductive tract prior to insemination facilitates the development of sensitization to spermatozoa and, in cattle so treated, the presence of high serum antibody titers has been associated with sterility. Currently, one of the greatest problems associated with attempts to correlate the titers of antisperm anibodies with infertility in both men and women is of a technological nature—assaying the antibodies (see Table 5-1). Sperm immobilization tests may give more meaningful results than sperm-agglutinating tests.

Table 5-1

Comparing various tests used to detect antibodies to human spermatozoa in serum, seminal plasma, or cervical mucus and the correlation of their results with infertility

Comments about tests	Macroscopic agglutination (Kibrick)	Immobilization	Micro-agglutination (Franklin-Dukes)	Immunofluorescence
Antibodies detected	IgG	IgG and IgM	None	IgG and IgM
Antigens responsible	Cell surface	Lactoferrin-sperm coating antigen	None	Sperm tail, acrosome, equatorial segment, and postnuclear cap
Complement dependent	No	Yes	No	No
Correlation with sterility in females	35%	18%	38%	Unknown
Positive response in controls	40%	0%	46%	Unknown
Correlation with sterility in males	3.3%	Unknown	Unknown	Unknown
Correlation with other tests	None	None	None	None

ANAPHYLACTIC REACTIVITY TO SEMEN

There are on record two thoroughly investigated cases of women in whom highly distressing, immediate-type allergic reactions consistently developed within minutes of sexual intercourse. The symptoms included cutaneous eruption and congestion of mucous membranes. In addition there was loss of consciousness and asthma in one of the cases. On the basis of skin tests and *in vitro* tests the antigen responsible was found to be associated with seminal plasma and not with spermatozoa, and it was present in the seminal plasma of *all* males tested (including some who had been vasectomized) suggesting that it was of prostatic or seminal vesicle origin. The antibody was of the reaginic (IgE) type. It will be recalled that this is the most recently described class of immunoglobulin and it has an affinity for surface receptors on mast cells and basophil leukocytes. Its reaction with antigen results in the release of a series of pharmacologically active mediators including histamine, slow reacting substance (SRS), and serotonin.

The rarity of this syndrome, which does of course indicate that the immunologic hazard associated with coitus is by no means entirely theoretical, is difficult to explain. Dr. Bernard Levine and his associates, of New York University School of Medicine, authors of one of the reports, suggest that a group of factors, both genetic and environmental, must occur together in a patient to permit the elicitation and expression of this dramatic, life-threatening reaction. These factors probably include ability to recognize the antigen, which is under the control of Ir genes, and the capacity to respond to the allergen presented at the mucosal membrane with the production of high avidity IgE antibody.

AUTOANTIGENIC STATUS OF SPERMATOZOA

Many studies have been conducted on the antigens associated with semen and of spermatozoa. We now know that human semen contains at least 16 identifiable antigens, 7 of which are present on spermatozoa (see Fig. 5-1), and the remainder are in the seminal plasma. Since 4 of the 7 sperm-associated antigens are also present in the plasma, they probably represent secondarily acquired antigens picked up by the sperms during exposure to various secretions as they pass through the male reproductive tract. Needless to say, the presence of these secondarily acquired "coating" antigens has impeded the identification of "native" cyto-specific sperm antigens.

In a classic study conducted in 1938 Drs. Henle, Henle, and Chambers at the University of Pennsylvania used ultrasound to separate the head from the tail of mouse sperms. By absorption analysis they were able to show that there was a head-specific as well as a tail-specific antigen, both of which were heat labile. In addition, there was a heat-stable, species-specific antigen present in both heads and tails. Three kinds of agglutination patterns exist for spermatozoa—head-to-head, tail-to-tail, or

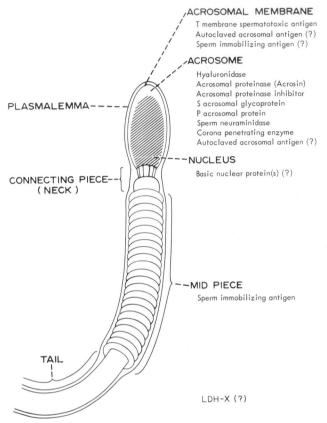

ACROSOMAL MEMBRANE
T membrane spermatotoxic antigen
Autoclaved acrosomal antigen (?)
Sperm immobilizing antigen (?)

ACROSOME
Hyaluronidase
Acrosomal proteinase (Acrosin)
Acrosomal proteinase inhibitor
S acrosomal glycoprotein
P acrosomal protein
Sperm neuraminidase
Corona penetrating enzyme
Autoclaved acrosomal antigen (?)

PLASMALEMMA

NUCLEUS
Basic nuclear protein(s) (?)

CONNECTING PIECE
(NECK)

MID PIECE
Sperm immobilizing antigen

TAIL

LDH-X (?)

Fig. 5-1. Schematic diagram of a human spermatozoon illustrating the morphologic localization of some of the antigens that are known to be associated with these highly specialized cells. Fluorescent antibody techniques have demonstrated some of these distinct antigens in the anterior portion of the head, the nucleus, the neck, and the midpiece as well as the tailpiece. Although numerous biochemically defined antigenic determinants are represented on spermatozoa, it appears that the midpiece "sperm-immobilizing" antigen is the one most likely to incite an immune response in the female that may lead to infertility. (From, J. S. Cochran. 1974. *Urology* 4:367–377.

neck-to-neck—indicating the restriction of specific surface antigenic determinants to these morphologic regions.

Toullet and her associates have fractionated epididymal spermatozoa of the guinea pig and studied them by a variety of immunological procedures. These have revealed the existence of 4 different antigens, designated S, P, Z, and T, having distinct locations and possessing the capacity to incite aspermatogenesis when inoculated together with CFA into guinea pigs. Each component seems to differ from the others both biochemically and antigenically as well as in its pathogenetic potency. Protein is associated with all of them. Chemical definition of these antigens is of the utmost importance from the viewpoint of immunopathology as well as from the viewpoint of those interested in immunologic contraception.

ALLOANTIGENIC STATUS OF SPERMATOZOA

Apart from the significance of the organ- or cyto-specific antigens associated with spermatozoa considered above, another important question in the immunobiology of mammalian reproduction is the extent to which the genetic determinants of cellular alloantigens express themselves in the phenotypes of sperms. Do spermatozoa only express antigens corresponding to their haploid genetic status, or does their cytoplasm continue to express all the antigens corresponding to their diploid precursor spermatogonial cells? In more practical terms, in spermatogenesis in an AB-type male, does a sperm carrying the allelic determinant for blood group A express only this antigen, or both the A and B antigens, and is there any evidence that sperms bearing the A allele are selected against by females of types B or O who have the corresponding alloantibody? In species such as mice and rats, in which there is a histocompatibility locus associated with the Y chromosome, do Y-bearing sperm express this specificity? The answers to these questions are still unclear, but the possibility that immunological forces of selection may be operating on sperm during their sojourn in the female reproductive tract is a very intriguing one that we shall consider in more detail later.

That antigens of the ABO blood group are expressed by sperm is attested by the results of a variety of different tests and was established as long ago as 1926 by Landsteiner and Levine. These cells can acquire blood group antigens secondarily by absorption from the seminal plasma of secretors. For example, group O sperm incubated with A secretor seminal plasma subsequently behave like spermatozoa from blood group A individuals. Whether the ABO antigens associated with human sperm are exclusively of secondary origin remains equivocal. Blood group antigens M, N, and Tja, although not present in seminal plasma, have also been identified on the sperm membrane. If we could detect Rh antigens on spermatozoa, it might enable us to separate the sperms from an Rh-positive Dd heterozygote into two populations. This would be extremely useful clinically to avoid situations in which an Rh-negative woman bears Rh-positive fetuses. Unfortunately, all attempts to detect these antigens on sperms have so far proved unsuccessful.

The demonstrability of antibodies to the ABO antigens in cervical mucus has raised the possibility that these antibodies might be capable of interacting with spermatozoa bearing the corresponding antigens and causing infertility. Studies on married couples infertile for no apparent cause, however, have failed to reveal any excess of ABO incompatible matings. Furthermore, by chance alone, one would expect about 20% of couples to be ABO incompatible and therefore infertile if these antibodies are of any significance, and this is certainly not the case. Thus ABO incompatibility acting at the level of the spermatozoa can only be a very infrequent cause of infertility.

Recently it has been shown that at least some transplantation antigens are also present on spermatozoa in mice, rats, hamsters, and men. In 1969 Vojtísková and her colleagues in Czechoslovakia succeeded in identifying some of the antigens determined by the H-2^d allele on mouse spermatozoa by means of a hemagglutinin absorption technique. Application of an indirect fluorescent antibody procedure to supensions of spermatozoa confirmed that these cells express antigenic specificities determined by the H-2 locus. In addition, experiments in which mice were inoculated intraperitoneally with allogeneic spermatozoa followed, 5-21 days later, by a test skin allograft of similar alien genetic origin, yielded suggestive evidence of the presence on sperm of antigens controlled by the linked minor H-3 and H-13 loci and by the H-Y male-specific locus. These workers were careful to point out that the sperm suspensions employed were obtained from the cauda epididymis and the vas deferens and were always contaminated by about 10% nonsperm cells. The presence of the latter might afford an alternative explanation for the results of both the hemagglutinin absorption and the grafting experiments. The findings with the immunofluorescent procedures were unequivocal, however, since the antigens were visualized directly and found to be associated with spermatozoa. Using a cytotoxicity test, Dr. Ellen Goldberg of Cornell University Medical College and co-workers have also demonstrated unequivocally that H-2 antigens are present on mouse spermatozoa.

In man, with the aid of specific HL-A tissue-typing sera and a microcytotoxicity test, Fellous and Dausset in Paris demonstrated that at least some of the specificities determined by the HL-A locus are present in high concentrations on sperm. When monospecific antiserum was employed to test sperms from donors known to be heterozygous for certain HL-A antigens, lysis of approximately 50% of the sperm population occurred, suggesting haploid expressions of the HL-A antigens. In other tests antigenically different types of sperm were detected in semen from a single donor. These latter findings are important since they minimize the possibility that the transplantation alloantigens expressed by sperm have been acquired by absorption from the seminal plasma. This work pioneers the way for genetic manipulation since pretreatment of sperm suspensions with an appropriate cytotoxic antibody could afford a means of selectively removing gametes carrying the determinant for a hereditary disease.

Gametic selection in dogs is being attempted by exposure of the sperms to anti-DL-A sera.

Encouraged by their evidence of the efficacy with which viable suspensions of lymphoid or epidermal cells inoculated via the intrauterine route sensitize animals against transplantation antigens, the present authors have studied the immunogenicity of allogeneic epididymal spermatozoa introduced by this route. Using different combinations of syngeneic strains of rats, mice, and hamsters, they have found that washed allogeneic sperms injected directly into the host's uterine lumen were as effective as similar numbers of lymph node cells in (1) stimulating hypertrophy of the draining, para-aortic lymph node and (2) sensitizing the host with respect to subsequent test skin allografts from the strain that donated the spermatozoa, transplanted 3 weeks later. It was also found that when C57BL/6 female mice received 10×10^6 sperms from males of their *own* strain (confronting them with the Y antigen), the majority rejected subsequent skin grafts from C57BL/6 males in an accelerated manner.

Previous observations by other workers that repeated mating of C57BL/6 females with males of their own strain, in the absence of pregnancy, caused some of the females to become incapable of rejecting syngeneic skin grafts from male donors also indicated the expression of the Y antigen by semen, probably by the spermatozoa.

Recently Beer and his associates have obtained evidence of cross-reactivity between the Y antigens of rats and mice. This comprised the discovery that inoculation of spermatozoa, but not lymphoid cells, from Fischer rats into the uteri of virgin C57BL/6 female mice caused them to reject subsequent grafts from C57BL/6 male donors in an accelerated manner.

If Syrian hamsters of the MHA strain that have been immunized against the tissue antigens of the unrelated CB strain are injected intradermally with viable cells, or antigenic extracts from CB donors, delayed tuberculin-like inflammatory reactions known as *direct hypersensitivity reactions* are evoked. Similar reactions can be evoked from female MHA hamsters that have previously been inoculated with CB hamster spermatozoa via the intrauterine route, indicating the presence of transplantation antigens on spermatozoa in this species too.

Careful appraisal of the proportion of contaminating nonsperm cells in the sperm suspensions that Beer and his co-workers used in their experiments, in conjunction with the comparatively small numbers of sperms in relatively pure suspensions (obtained by differential centrifugation) required to immunize against skin allografts, made it seem unlikely that the presence of contaminating nonspermatozoal cells were responsible for the apparent immunogenicity. This conclusion was reinforced by the finding that doses of spermatozoa found to be effective in eliciting transplantation immunity when injected into the uterus proved to be completely ineffective when administered by other routes, including the foot pads.

The fact that repeated normal matings did not elicit sensitization on the part of female hosts hinted that either the numbers of sperm gaining entrance to the uterus at any one time remained a subthreshold stimulus or that these cells were cleared very rapidly from this organ.

LOCAL ANTIBODY PRODUCTION IN THE UTERUS

There have been few attempts to study the immunological activity of physiological uterotubal secretions of subjects immunized primarily by the intrauterine route. The uterine endometrium of most higher mammals is abundantly endowed with lymphatics and seems to have all the prerequisites to deliver either antigen, or antigen-primed—i.e., peripherally sensitized—immunologically competent cells of hematologic origin, as well as macrophages, to a draining lymph node. Diffuse deposits of lymphoid cells beneath the endometrium may be triggered to produce antibody (very probably IgA) locally that may be transported across the mucous membrane and into lumen. Available evidence hints, however, that the local production of antibody at the uterine level against seminal antigens is minimal when serum antibody levels in the same individual are taken into consideration. The suggestion has been made that one of the functions of IgA antibodies may be to prevent harmful antigens from gaining entry to the body by forming nonabsorbable stable complexes with them.

It is pertinent to mention here that a great deal of attention has been focused on the general arrangement of the lymphatic vessels in the uterine wall and their ultimate drainage into the lumbar lymph nodes, principally in order to follow the pathways in puerperal sepsis and the metastatic spread of endometrial carcinoma in the uterus. During pregnancy in all species, the main lymphatic plexuses, which are situated between the inner circular and the outer longitudinal muscles, become greatly increased in size but not in number. There is evidence that the development of these uterine vessels, at various stages of pregnancy, runs parallel with the need to remove increasing amounts of tissue fluid. The demonstration that uterine venous blood is more concentrated than arterial blood suggested a high filtration rate with a high rate of lymph formation.

It has been suggested that in males, in addition to the blood-testis barrier, another safeguard that may help prevent autoimmunization if "self" antigenic constituents are accidentally released is their prompt inactivation at the site by enzymes known to exist in the reproductive organs and sera. Katsh has produced evidence in support of this thesis and suggested that deficiency in one or more of these enyzmatic degradation systems might allow an autoimmune response to be stimulated.

Disposal of coitally inoculated antigens is a problem confronting females. Soluble substances may undergo absorption through the mucosa of the genital tract. Spermatozoa may be lost in part through their penetration of the lining of the epithelium of the genital tract, but phagocytosis by macrophages is probably the principal process responsible for their removal. Katsh has shown that in the guinea pig both serum and uterine tissue extract contains enzymes capable of inactivating the aspermatogenic antigen.

SOMATIC FERTILIZATION

The demonstration, by Terni and Maleci in 1937, that living rooster spermatozoa can penetrate living chicken embryonic cells *in vitro* stimulated considerable interest in somatic fertilization and its possible immunological consequences. The heads of spermatozoa have been found in epithelial cells of the Fallopian tube in several different species of rodents leading to the conclusion, on the basis of the frequency and reproducibility of these observations, that this phenomenon is widespread. The potential significance of this process has been underscored by Reid and Blackwell's evidence of incorporation of material from the labeled nuclei of living mouse sperm by peritoneal macrophages with which they had been maintained *in vitro* for 17 hours. Particularly pertinent is evidence that blood group A human sperm cultured with type O Hela cells were capable of passing the A antigen on to the latter. The mechanism by which the cultured cells acquired their new antigen, and its persistence, has yet to be elucidated. If somatic fertilization is a common event *in vivo* and if spermatozoa are able to transmit, even transiently, genetically usable "information" to their host cells, then the apparent potent immunogenicity of homologous sperm when introduced into the uterine cavity of rodents may be partially explained.

R E F E R E N C E S

Ansbacher, R., Yeung, K. K., and Behrman, S. J. 1973. "Clinical significance of sperm antibodies in infertile couples." *Fertil. Steril.* **24**:305–308.

Beer, A. E., and Billingham, R. E. 1974. "Host responses to intrauterine tissue, cellular and fetal allografts." *J. Reprod. Fertil. Suppl.* **21**:59–88.

76   THE ANTIGENIC STATUS OF SEMEN

Behrman, S. J., and Menge, A. C. 1972. "Immunologic role of seminal antigens in fertility control." In *Control of human fertility physiological mechanisms and clinical applications* (T. N. Evans and E. S. E. Hafez, ed.). Harper and Row, New York.

Bell, E. B., and McLaren, A. 1970. "Reduction of fertility in female mice iso-immunized with a sub-cellular sperm fraction." *J. Reprod. Fertil.* **22**:345–356.

Boettcher, B. 1974. "The molecular nature of sperm-agglutinins and sperm antibody in human sera." *J. Reprod. Fertil. Suppl.* **22**:151–167.

Fellous, M., and Dausset, J. 1970. "Probable haploid expression of the HL-A antigens on human spermatozoon." *Nature* **225**:191–193.

Goldberg, E. H., Boyse, E. A., Bennett, D., Scheid, M., and Carswell, E. A. 1971. "Serological demonstration of H-Y (male) antigen on mouse sperm." *Nature* **232**:478–480.

Halpern, B. N., Ky, T., and Robert, B. 1967. "Clinical and immunological study of an exceptional case of reaginic type sensitization to human seminal fluid." *Immunology* **12**:247–258.

Katsh, S. 1959. "Immunology, fertility and infertility: A historical survey." *Am. J. Obstet Gynecol.* **77**:946–956.

Katsh, S. 1969. "Immunological aspects of reproduction." *In Ovum implantation* (M. C. Shelesnyak and G. J. Marcus, ed.). Gordon and Breach, New York, pp. 309–344.

Levine, B. B., Siraganian, R. P., and Schenkein, I. 1973. "Allergy to human seminal plasma." *N. Eng. J. Med.* **288**:894–896.

McLaren, A. 1966. "Studies on the isoimmunization of mice with spermatozoa." *Fertil. Steril.* 17:492–499.

Reid, B. L., and Blackwell, P. M. 1967. "Evidence for the possibility of nuclear uptake of polymerised deoxyribonucleic acid of sperm phagocytosed by macrophages." *Austral. J. Exp. Biol. Med. Sci.* **45**:323–326.

Rümke, Ph. 1968. "The spermatozoa and testes in allergic disease." In *Clinical aspects of immunology* (P. G. H. Gell and R. R. A. Coombs, ed.). Blackwell, Oxford, pp. 1143–1159.

Terni, T., and Maleci, O. 1937. "Über das Eindringen von Spermatozoen in in-vitro gezüchtete somatische Zellen." *Arch. f. exper. Zellforsch.* **19**:165–170.

Vojtíšková, M. 1969. "H-2d antigens on mouse spermatozoa." *Nature* **222**:1293–1294.

Chapter 6

The Fetus as an Allograft:
Consideration of Some of the Factors
That May Contribute to Its Success

With the growth of knowledge concerning the immunogenetic factors that curtail the survival of tumor, normal tissue, and organ grafts exchanged between members of outbred populations or different inbred or syngeneic strains, and of the peremptory rejection of "second-set" allografts by sensitized hosts, came recognition that the feto-placental unit, as an almost invariably successful allograft, occupies a paradoxical position. The fundamental principle that grafts from an F_1 hybrid donor are rejected when transplanted to either of its parents obviously does not apply to "naturally transplanted" F_1 hybrid conceptuses during their development in the maternal uterus.

The classic experiment that established the transferability of fertilized eggs also represented the first experimental investigation of the fetal allograft problem. In 1891 Walter Heape, in London, transferred two fertilized Angora rabbit eggs from a doe, mated to an Angora buck 32 hours beforehand, to the fallopian tube of a Belgian hare that had been mated 3 hours previously with a male of her own breed (see Fig. 6-1). The subsequent birth of a litter comprising four Belgian hares and two Angoras afforded formal proof that fetuses require no genetic endowment from their mothers (in the form of a haploid set of chromosomes) in order to survive to term. Subsequent investigators have established the invulnerability to rejection of transferred immunogenetically alien zygotes in a wide range of species that includes mice, rats, guinea pigs, rabbits, cattle, and sheep.

Repeated attempts have been made to prejudice implantation and normal development *in utero* to term of conceptuses resulting from heterospecific matings (i.e., matings between genetically dissimilar parents) in mice, rats, guinea pigs and rabbits, etc., by presensitization or adoptive immunization of the mothers against the alien, paternally inherited transplantation antigens of their fetuses. In no instance have these measures

77

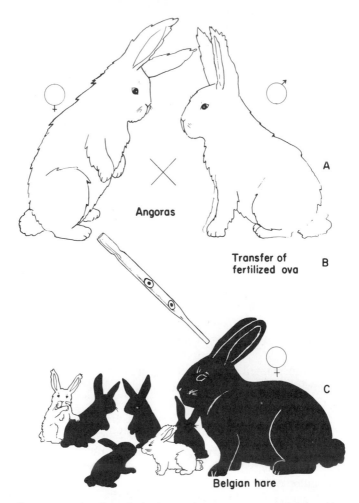

Fig. 6-1. Illustrating Walter Heape's classic experiment on ovum transfer in rabbits. Two Angoras were mated (A) and two of the resultant fertilized eggs (B) transferred to the fallopian tube of a Belgian hare (C) that had been mated to a male of her own breed. Subsequently this animal gave birth to a litter of six young—four Belgian hares and two Angoras.

succeeded—live healthy babies have consistently been delivered. Particularly forceful evidence of the futility of such attempts was the failure on the part of Dr. Jonathan Lanman and his associates to impair the development to term of blastocysts transferred to the uteri of pseudo-pregnant female rabbits *hyperimmunized,* by means of skin allografts, against the tissue antigens of *both* parents of the transferred zygotes (the three rabbits involved in each experiment were genetically disparate). The presence of high titers of cytotoxic antibodies in the maternal blood had no deleterious influence on the fetuses, although the latter sometimes acquired these antibodies from the maternal circulation. Indeed, in Lanman's experiments antibody was demonstrable in the blastocoele fluid.

It is important to note, however, that there is one observation that differs from those summarized above. Drs. Breyere and Sprenger of the American University in Washington, D.C., hyperimmunized C57 BL female mice against DBA or C3H strain tissue antigens by means of repeated inoculations of allogeneic tumor cells. The immunized females were then mated with males of one or the other of these strains. They observed a 6–16% reduction in the number of F_1 hybrid offspring delivered by specifically immunized females as compared with those delivered by the nonspecifically immunized, or unimmunized, females (i.e., controls). These authors put forward the intriguing suggestion that the variance of their findings with those of other workers might be due to the sharing of an antigen by both the fetal and the tumor tissues that was absent in normal adult tissue. Further study is needed to determine the stage in development at which elimination of the conceptuses occurred or indeed whether such a process took place, for it is conceivable that the immunity was effective against the spermatozoa *before* fertilization.

Many hypotheses have been advanced to account for the success of fetuses as allografts, the more important of which we shall now consider in relation to the evidence that bears upon them (see Fig. 6-2). It will be recalled that one of these hypotheses—that the uterus represents an immunologically privileged site—has already been dealt with and dismissed as being capable, at best, of affording only a very marginal degree of protection to a fetus in an unsensitized mother and no protection whatsoever in specifically sensitized mothers (see Chapter 2). Another hypothesis, that there is an alteration in the maternal capacity to undertake or express immunological reactions during pregnancy, will be considered in the following chapter.

COMPLETE SEPARATION OF MATERNAL AND FETAL CIRCULATIONS

Despite the fact that the complexity and the intimacy of the interface between maternal and fetal tissues at the level of the placenta display a wide range of structural variations between species—the basis of comparative placentology—fetal and maternal circulations are always *completely* separate. Apart from its possible physiological significance, this separation has long been regarded as a critically important protective factor from the immunologic viewpoint. Breakdown of this vascular quarantine would clearly lead to sensitization of the mother against a multiplicity of isoantigens associated with both cellular and other components of the fetal blood and provide ready access of the resultant antibodies and specific lymphocytic effector cells to the fetal circulation. Apart from

(A) ANATOMICAL LEVELS AT WHICH MATERNAL IMMUNOCYTES MAY ENCOUNTER AND INTERACT WITH CELLS OF THE FETUS

MATERNAL REGIONAL LYMPH NODES AND SPLEEN   TROPHOBLASTIC-DECIDUAL FRONTIER   LYMPHOMYELOID COMPLEX AND SKIN OF THE FETUS

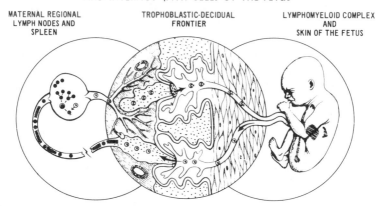

(B) THEORIES PROPOUNDED TO ACCOUNT FOR THE INVULNERABILITY OF THE FETO-PLACENTAL UNIT TO REJECTION

ALTERED IMMUNOLOGICAL RESPONSIVENESS OF MOTHER	UTERUS	TROPHOBLAST	FETUS
Non-Specific	1. Complete Separation of Fetal and Maternal Circulations	1. Non Antigenic	1. Antigenic Immaturity
1. Placental Protein or Steroid Hormones		2. Physiologic Barrier	
2. Plasma Factors		3. Local Immunosuppression by Hormones (HCG and HCS)	2. Serum Factors (fetuin)
Specific	2. Immunologically Privileged Site (decidual tissue)		
1. Antibody Mediated .Suppression			
2. Adult Tolerance			

Fig. 6-2. Illustrating the major anatomical components of the maternal-fetal relationship and summarizing the principal known or suggested factors that may account for the consistent non-rejection of the fetus as an allograft. The right-hand circle presents the fetus freely suspended in the fluid in the amniotic sac cavity and connected via the paired umbilical arteries and vein to the sustaining placenta (center circle). The left-hand circle represents the maternal uterus with its draining para-aortic lymph nodes. The center circle represents the organ of exchange between the mother and fetus—the placenta—in which there is a continuous unbroken frontier of epithelial tissue of fetal origin—the trophoblast—directly and intimately juxtaposed to maternal uterine decidual tissue or to maternal blood in the intervillus spaces. Although there are no direct interconnections between the blood circulations of the fetus and its mother, the trophoblast is permeable to cells that may cross it in either direction.

the possibility of these cells inducing a state of tolerance of maternal antigens in their immature hosts, some of them would certainly be expected to react against alien cellular antigens of their hosts, causing runt or graft-versus-host disease. A model of the possible disastrous consequences of free, maternal-fetal vascular intercommunication is afforded by the phenomenon of *parabiosis intoxication*. This is best studied in situations in which parental strain individuals are surgically parabiosed to their F_1 hybrids; the latter become "intoxicated." The clinical picture in this homologous or transplantation disease syndrome is still incompletely understood, being complicated by a shunting of blood from the F_1 to its parental strain partner, leading to anemia and polycythemia, respectively. However, graft-versus-host reactivity *within* the victim on the part of transferred immunologically competent cells from the parental strain individual both initiates and makes an important contribution to the disease, which is usually fatal.

To explore the effects of establishing direct vascular connections between mothers and fetuses, and so bypassing the placental barrier, Dr. B. T. Jackson ingeniously implanted maternal omentum beneath the skins of dog and sheep fetuses *in utero*. This resulted in the deaths of the fetal puppies within 2-3 days and those of the fetal lambs within 3-10 days. Pathological findings in the dying fetuses included generalized edema, hemorrhages into major organs, and occasional though not very conspicuous cell infiltrates. That these deaths were due to an immunologic response on the part of the mother or to a variant of the parabiosis intoxication syndrome now seems highly improbable in the light of Dr. James Scott's and his associates' recent observations that a similar, fatal disease afflicts rabbit, rat, and guinea pig fetuses that are *syngeneic* with their mothers, after this surgical procedure has established direct maternal-fetal vascular intercommunication. Here the evidence is very compelling that the marked polycythemia and early death of the subjects were due to circulatory overload and other disturbances of a physiological nature.

In striking contrast to the evident dangers of maternal-fetal vascular intercommunication is the apparent harmlessness of the synchorial vascular anastomoses that are consistently established between multiple fetuses in cattle and marmosets and rarely in man and sheep, irrespective of whether the fetuses concerned are genetically similar or dissimilar (see Chapter 10).

Lack of vascular connections with their maternal hosts cannot explain either the apparent inability of fetuses to elicit transplantation immunity in their mothers or their resistance to it. This is evidenced by observations that when allografts of pure epidermis or corneal epithelium are transplanted to extensive wound beds prepared by removal of the entire thickness of the skin of guinea pigs and rabbits, an immune response is incited in the host as a consequence of which the grafts are destroyed in a typical manner, despite the fact that they are never penetrated by blood vessels.

ANTIGENIC IMMATURITY OF THE FETUS EXEMPTS IT FROM REJECTION: ONTOGENY OF TRANSPLANTATION ANTIGENS

In 1924 Dr. C. C. Little put forward the ingenious suggestion that "the embryo has no definite physiologic characteristics which are individual enough to be recognized as foreign to the mother." This notion was soon placed in jeopardy by early observations that minced embryonic tissue allografts implanted into adult hosts are highly effective in eliciting immunity to subsequent test allografts of tumor or skin having the same genetic makeup as the immunizing fetal tissue grafts. Such findings were indecisive, however, in the sense that they failed to exclude the possibility of antigenic maturation or differentiation on the part of the fetal tissue allografts subsequent to their transplantation. More critical studies have minimized or obviated this possible complication in a variety of ways, which include (1) restriction of the time available for the embryonic cells to sensitize their hosts, by transplantation of embryonic tissue grafts to presensitized hosts and studying the cellular response a few days later; (2) preclusion of further differentiation of the embryonic cells used as antigen by irradiation; (3) evaluation of the capacity of embryonic cells to induce tolerance in infant hosts whose own age is such that their ability to become tolerant following inoculation with relatively small numbers of cells has almost disappeared; (4) determination of the ability of embryonic cell preparations to absorb specific alloantibodies, usually by hemagglutination inhibition; (5) direct visualization of the antigenic sites on cells by fluorescent antibody procedures or by indirect erythrocyte "rosette" procedures (in these tests the antigens recognized may not be transplantation antigens); and finally (6) determination of the capacity of alloimmune serum in the presence of complement to impair the development *in vitro* of mouse tubal eggs from which the zona pellucida has been removed.

The results of the studies that have been performed upon mice may be summarized as follows: Transplantation antigens appear very early in ontogeny, as evidenced, for example, by the failure of allogenic two- to eight-cell pretrophoblastic tubal eggs to develop into small trophoblastic tumors following implantation beneath the renal capsules of specifically hyperimmunized hosts or by their failure to develop further after explantation *in vitro* in the presence of alloantibody and complement. Discriminating immunofluorescence and other *in vitro* studies have confirmed the presence of antigens corresponding to so-called minor histocompatibility loci, including H-3, H-6, and H-13, distributed over the entire surface of the blastomeres of early two- to eight-cell preimplantation zygotes. Presently available evidence suggests that H-2 determined specificities are lacking from eggs. It is interesting to compare the apparent absence of H-2 determinants on early egg stages with their unequivocal presence on spermatozoa. Conceivably this reflects the more favorable opportunity enjoyed by the latter to absorb H-2 substances from their fluid milieu during maturation and storage.

Although grafting tests performed with blastocysts—i.e., 3½ to 4½-day embryos—indicate the presence of H-2 determinants at this stage, serological tests, which may be less sensitive, have failed to corroborate this. In carefully designed and well-controlled experiments using congenic resistant strains of mice differing only at the H-2 locus and using the cellular response of specifically presensitized hosts to grafts of embryonic tissue freed from ectoplacental cone material as an indication of host response, Dr. H. L. Patthey has obtained evidence of the appearance of H-2 specificities in a form capable of inciting the expression of an extant cellular immunity between the sixth and seventh days of development. Grafting and other studies conducted upon older murine embryos leave no doubt as to their expression of transplantation antigens but the majority of the tests were incapable of revealing whether specificities present correspond to major or minor histocompatibility loci.

Dr. Michael Schlesinger's careful quantitative absorption studies with a hemagglutinating antiserum established the presence of H-2 specificities in 10½-day embryos, and both he and other workers have shown that the antigen content of fetal liver increases progressively between 10½ days of gestation and term. Other serologic investigations on midterm or older fetuses have nearly all attested to the presence of both H-2 and other H antigens and indicated that the density of these antigens on the cell surfaces increases progressively toward term. In both spleen cells and erythrocytes a rapid increase in H-2 antigen concentration takes place during the first few days after birth. There is also evidence that not all the multiplicity of specificities determined by the H-2 locus mature at the same rate.

Grafting tests conducted upon both fetal and perinatal liver, heart, and skin allografts have yielded results consistent with the thesis that antigenic maturation is a progressive process that is not complete at delivery —such grafts live much longer than comparable grafts from adult donors.

With other species of mammals there is a dearth of precise information on the time of appearance and qualitative and quantitative aspects of the development of transplantation antigens. Histological studies on fetal tissues grafted to mothers specifically presensitized against paternal tissue antigens have indicated the presence of transplantation antigens in 15-day-old rat and 16-day-old rabbit fetuses. In both rabbits and hamsters, skin allografts from infant donors may long outlive grafts from adult donors.

Three approaches have been adopted to study the ontogeny of HL-A antigens in man: (1) explantation of various fetal tissues *in vitro* for various periods before the resultant outgrowing cells, mainly fibroblasts, were subjected to a mixed agglutination test, (2) direct typing of cells from fetuses by the fluorochromatic cytotoxicity test, and (3) study of the material solubilized and released from freshly obtained fetal tissues by ultrasonication. The first approach is, of course, complicated by the possibility of antigenic maturation of the cells during culture. The findings indicate that HL-A antigens are present on some cell types as early as 6–10 weeks and are probably present on all tissues by about 5 months.

Clearly much more work has to be done to clarify the situation, and the likelihood is that more discriminating tests will establish the expression of these specificities much earlier in development.

The overall conclusion to be drawn from these studies on the ontogeny of transplantation antigens is that these antigens are present in immunologically effective concentrations on the tissues of embryos from a very early stage, i.e., that these tissues are capable of eliciting transplantation immunity and are suspectible to it, and that the density of antigenic determinant sites increases with age, even after birth in some species, and at different rates in some tissues. Obviously, of much greater relevance to our understanding of the anomalous behavior of the fetus as an allograft is the antigenic status of its *extraembryonic* tissues—comprised of the fetal membranes, the yolk sac, and (above all) the placenta, especially its trophoblastic component. The latter represents the frontier where tissue of fetal origin is intimately juxtaposed to maternal tissue over a considerable surface area—up to 15 square meters in 20-week fetuses in man.

ALLOANTIGENICITY OF THE TROPHOBLAST

Several ingenious attempts have been made to account for the apparent lack of alloantigenicity of the trophoblast. In 1960 Gordon postulated that the outer layer of this epithelial tissue—the syncytial trophoblast, which is in direct contact with maternal tissue—develops from *maternal* cells of the ovarian follicle rather than from the implanting, fertilized egg. However, this interpretation disregards a great deal of embryological evidence. Also in 1960, the late Dr. Michael Galton of Dartmouth College suggested, on the basis of cytologic evidence (the presence or absence of Barr bodies, indicative of the presence of XX chromosomes), that syncytiotrophoblast is haploid, being derived from the zygote's *maternal* set of chromosomes. Compelling evidence that syncytiotrophoblast arises by differentiation from cytotrophoblast rather than by any unique kind of mitotic activity has refuted this premise.

An observation that does allow for speculation as to how trophoblast might undergo some kind of modification in response to its maternal environment is that during the implantation of blastocysts in both rabbits and mice the plasma membranes of trophoblast and maternal decidual cells fuse and break down. Does this facilitate an exchange of cytoplasmic materials? It has been shown in several species that the syncytiotrophoblast nuclei contain 500–1000 times the haploid amount of DNA. Three possible mechanisms could explain this phenomenon: (1) endomitosis resulting in the formation of polytene or polyploid chromosomes; (2) uptake of maternal nuclei or molecular DNA as the trophoblast invades the endometrium; or (3) the syncytiotrophoblast may form by cell fusion, followed by subsequent fusion of the nuclei. Drs. Gearhart and Mintz, working with mouse strains of differing isoenzyme variants, transferred GPI-1A strain fertilized eggs to GPI-1B foster mothers. They found no evidence of heteropolymer (GPI-1AB) isozyme in the trophoblast from these transferred embryos, indicating that the trophoblast does not functionally incorporate maternal DNA nor does it form syncytial heterokaryons by cell fusion. It appears more likely that the increased DNA content of trophoblast cells results from endomitosis leading to polyploidy. These investigators also showed that trophoblast giant cell formation was not induced by the uterine environment at the time of implantation but was a function intrinsic to the trophoblast, for nuclei with 4X haploid amount of DNA were detected prior to implantation.

Any theory that ascribes the success of fetuses as allografts to absence of paternally inherited alloantigens in syncytiotrophoblast is utterly and decisively discredited by the high degree of success of allogeneic zygote transfers to normal or even to presensitized surrogate mothers.

Although many grafting experiments have been conducted with placental tissue, or with cell suspensions prepared therefrom, their design has been too crude to be very informative. These tests have usually entailed grafting placental tissue, or suspensions of cells obtained from them, to normal host mice of the *maternal* strain so that contaminating cells of maternal origin were incapable of provoking sensitivity. This approach has certainly established that (1) paternally inherited transplantation antigens are present in the placenta, possibly associated with contaminating fetal leukocytes or "passenger" cells, and (2) F_1 hybrid placental grafts are vulnerable to rejection in maternal strain hosts presensitized against the tissue antigens of the paternal strain. At least some components of this ephemeral organ of composite histological makeup are thus susceptible to destruction.

Physiological Barrier Between Mother and Fetus

The most striking quality of the fetus as an organismic allograft *in utero* is its apparent total refractoriness to a state of immunity or hyperimmunity on the part of its maternal host directed against its own transplantation antigens. This resistant property—a form of efferent inhibition of the immune response—is expressed most dramatically in species with hemochorial placentas, where maternal blood, which bears both antigen-sensitive lymphocytes as well as effector or "killer" lymphocytes in the case of sensitized animals, is continuously in contact with a large area of fetal trophoblast cells (see Fig. 1-4).

Only one hypothesis can reasonably account for the survival to term of fetuses in both normal and sensitized mothers and the various observations presented so far—i.e., fetuses are surrounded by some kind of physical or anatomical barrier capable of (1) preventing the mother from developing a state of transplantation immunity to the alien histo-compatibility antigens of her fetuses and (2) affording the latter complete protection against high levels of sensitivity procured by prior grafting with normal tissues of appropriate alien genetic origin or by adoptive immunization.

Simply because it represents the continuous, uninterrupted "frontier" component of the fetus, the trophoblast came under suspicion as fulfilling this role. As we've seen already, the anatomic complexity of the maternal-fetal relationship in the placenta, which is determined principally by the precisely ordered invasiveness of the trophoblast into maternal decidual tissue, varies widely from species to species. It ranges from a simple close apposition of trophoblast to the intact endometrial epithelium of the uterus found in pigs and horses to an erosive penetration of trophoblastic tissue through the endometrial epithelium, its subjacent connective tissue, blood vessel walls, and even the endothelium of maternal veins so that fetal trophoblast cells covering the trophoblastic villi come into direct contact with and are actually bathed by maternal blood as in the hemo-chorial placentas of humans, rodents, and rabbits (see Chapter 1).

INCRIMINATION OF TROPHOBLAST AS
THE QUARANTINING LAYER

In 1928 the late Dr. Ernest Witebsky and his associates discovered that human placental villi are deficient in blood group antigens, an observation that has subsequently been confirmed by an immunofluorescence technique. On the basis of their observation, the Witebsky group explicitly suggested that placenta could function as an immunological protective barrier if its trophoblast cells were nonantigenic. In 1959 Drs. W. A. Bardawil and B. L. Toy suggested an alternative, trophoblast-associated candidate to fulfill the role of sequestration—the *layer of Nitabuch,* a local zone of fibrinoid substance, probably a degeneration product of both trophoblast and decidua that in man normally separates maternal and fetal tissue where invading trophoblast meets decidual tissue. Bardawil and Toy proposed that this layer might behave "as an immunological no man's land, walling the fetus off from chemical interaction with its host."

The success of choriocarcinoma of gestational origin as a foreign tumor graft has long been interpreted as reflecting the lack of alloantigenicity of its normal tissue of origin—cytotrophoblast. Indeed, this is probably the only example of a tumor that has shed some light upon an important, distinctive feature of its normal precursor tissue. Finally, the development of human and other fetuses for long periods and occasionally to term, in a variety of nonuterine ectopic sites, such as the fallopian tubes, the ileum and rectum, and the peritoneum affords compelling evidence that whatever is responsible for the immunological quarantining layer must be of fetal origin and highly versatile with regard to its capacity for functional deployment. Reports on ectopic pregnancies provide no grounds for suspicion that immunologic reactivity on the part of the mother plays a causal role in fetal death under these circumstances.

TRANSPLANTATION STUDIES ON TROPHOBLAST

For the first discriminating analysis of the histocompatibility properties of mouse placental tissue we are indebted to Drs. Richard Simmons and Paul S. Russell who studied grafts of allogeneic mouse placental tissue at various stages of its development. In most of their experiments, grafts from F_1 hybrid embryos were transplanted to hosts of the maternal strain to exclude the possibility of sensitization of the host by contaminating maternal tissue fragments and cells.

Initially they confirmed the findings of others that allografts of placenta from 10½-day embryos elicited and succumbed to a typical host response, whether implanted intramuscularly or to host sites prepared in the skin. Then, recognizing the difficulty of interpreting the results of this kind of experiment in which the graft was comprised of several cell types, they took advantage of the separability of 7½-day mouse embryos into trophoblastic precursors (the ectoplacental cone) and the embryo itself. When transplanted beneath the renal capsules of maternal strain hosts that had been presensitized against the tissue antigens of the paternal strain, the embryonic grafts were totally destroyed within 7 days. The trophoblastic tissue allografts underwent marked proliferative activity, however, on the part of their giant cells, which, by their phagocytic and invasive activities, formed typical blood spaces in the host renal parenchyma. Furthermore, there was little cellular response against these grafts on the part of the host. These trophoblastic allografts underwent a sort of nonspecific involution after 12-13 days, just as they did when placed in genetically compatible hosts. Any trophoblastic cells accidentally included in embryonic grafts transplanted to sensitized hosts behaved as if completely unaffected by the cell-mediated destructive process that destroyed their nontrophoblastic neighbors.

When two- to eight-cell stage fertilized eggs were harvested from the fallopian tubes and transplanted ectopically beneath the renal capsules or into the spleens of syngeneic hosts, a significant proportion of these developed into small tumors of trophoblastic giant cells, displaying invasive properties and having a finite life-span of about 14 days. When F_1 hybrid ova of this early developmental age were placed in the kidneys of un-immunized hosts of the maternal strain, their life-span underwent no curtailment nor did the host become immunized to the tissue antigens of the donor strain. More impressive was the continued survival and tran-sient growth of these pure trophoblastic allografts in hosts presensitized by means of two consecutive skin allografts from the paternal strain.

Further supportive evidence of the competence of trophoblast to pro-vide an effective immunologic buffer zone for the fetus derived from com-parative studies on the fates of allogeneic two- to eight-cell tubal eggs, $3\frac{1}{2}$-day blastocysts, and ectoplacental cones from 7-day allogeneic em-bryos transplanted to specifically hypersensitized H-2 locus-incompatible murine hosts. The proportion of eggs transplanted beneath the renal cap-sules of alien male mice, presensitized to various degrees against donor strain tissue antigens, that developed into trophoblastic tissue was found to be inversely related to the level of immunity in the host. For example, trophoblast failed to develop in hosts sensitized by two consecutive skin allografts followed by 8-12 injections of spleen cells. F_1 hybrid eggs proved to be less susceptible in similar hyperimmune hosts, however, probably because of a gene-dosage effect—the hybrid cells having fewer alien de-terminant sites on their membranes. In all instances in which trophoblastic proliferation occurred in these hyperimmune hosts, its extent was not demonstrably curtailed.

In contradistinction to the vulnerability of ectopically transplanted fertilized eggs in hyperimmunized hosts, ectoplacental cone grafts from 7 day embryos proved to be completely refractory. On the basis of these observations, Simmons and Russell drew the interesting conclusion that transplantation antigens are present in the pretrophoblastic embryo, but the trophoblast represents a functionally specialized form of embryonic cell that is incapable of manufacturing or expressing on its surface antigens displayed by its immediate precursors. It is interesting to note that when allogeneic blastocysts were transplanted orthotopically to the uteri instead of beneath the renal capsules of pseudopregnant hyperimmune females, there was no impairment of development. Two possible explanations for this differential viability of the allogeneic blastocysts in the two sites are (1) the surrounding decidual tissue in the uterus afforded them some degree of protection—this seems rather unlikely in the light of some of the present authors' findings (see page 24)—or (2) through some kind of interaction between decidual tissue and trophoectoderm the latter acquires its immunologic protective properties prematurely.

INTERSPECIFIC HYBRIDS AND XENOGENEIC FETUSES

It is generally agreed that the histocompatibility barriers that exist when graft donor and host are members of *different* species (i.e., xenografts) are usually much greater than those present where allografts are involved. The evidence sustaining this generalization, of course, is the curtailment of survival times of xenografts as compared with that of allografts. The birth of healthy interspecific hybrids after matings between horses and donkeys, possibly sheep and goats, leopards and tigers; cattle, bison and yak in different combinations; and bears of different species affords *prima facie* evidence of the considerable potential of the trophoblast to override histocompatibility barriers.

The difficulties in obtaining live-born interspecific hybrids are believed to be attributable to (1) the presence of alien, potent *species-specific* antigens associated with the spermatozoa, the seminal plasma, and the membranes of the conceptus; (2) differences between the karyotypes of the two parent species, leading to problems of mitosis, etc.; and (3) immunologic reactivity on the part of the mother against foreign, species-specific cellular antigens of the hybrid fetus and its membranes, notably its trophoblast.

When female goats are inseminated with sheep semen, conception readily occurs but the hybrid embryos usually die at about the end of the sixth week of gestation. In most workers' experience the reciprocal mating is unsuccessful. Dr. K. Bratanov and his colleagues in Bulgaria have claimed, however, that in sheep the chances of fertilization are increased by repeated insemination of anestrous ewes with goat semen before the effective insemination or by pretreatment of the goat spermatozoa with ram seminal plasma.

Ultrastructural studies on the placentas of 34- to 38-day goat × sheep hybrid embryos from pregnant goats, by Dr. Jennifer Dent and co-workers of the Royal Veterinary College in London, revealed endothelial damage and platelet accumulations in maternal uterine subepithelial vessels as well as damage to the epithelium, but no damage to the trophoblast. These and other findings suggest that the lesions may have been caused by antigen-antibody complexes, supporting the reasonable contention that death of the hybrids in this combination has an immunological basis.

Female ferrets (*Mustela furo*) have been successfully inseminated with mink (*Mustela vision*) sperm and evidence of massive hemorrhage at the placental sites of 2-week embryos has been obtained. There are thus good grounds for belief that in the case of interspecific hybrids maternal immunologic reactivity against the fetuses precludes the delivery of live offspring in many different combinations.

When fertilized eggs are transferred across species barriers factors 1 and 2 are eliminated, but factor 3 remains and may even be exacerbated as a consequence of a gene dosage effect. To date relatively few extensive investigations have been performed on the survival potential of interspecifically transferred blastocysts. With certain species combinations, it has been shown that xenografts of trophoblastic tissue survive, displaying typical mitotic-proliferative properties. Although rat eggs display only feeble development following insertion beneath the renal capsules of mice, upward of 25% of mouse eggs placed in the kidneys of rat hosts produce flourishing trophoblastic tissue that invades and phagocytizes its host milieu just as it would have done in a host of its own species. However, 6½-day mouse embryos divested of their trophoblastic moiety and transplanted to rat kidneys incite massive cellular responses. Mouse trophoblast is able to grow in the testes of rats and hamsters; hamster trophoblast will grow in mice; and in none of these combinations has there been evidence of a host immunological response. The observation that the growth of mouse ectoplacental cone grafts inserted beneath the testicular capsules of rats was inhibited if the hosts had previously been grafted with mouse skin suggests that species-specific antigens are expressed by trophoblast.

Drs. Kirby and Tarkowski have transferred rat blastocysts into ovariectomized mice rendered pseudopregnant by injection of progesterone, delayed implantation for 2–3 days by further administration of progesterone, and followed this by injection of estrogen to induce implantation. Under these conditions, implantation of some of the embryos occurred and some developed into completely normal rat fetuses that died around the fourteenth day of development, possibly because of size limitation. The placentas of these fetuses remained viable and persisted almost to term. The prospects of obtaining longer survivals with the mouse-to-rat combination seem much better, although this has apparently not yet been attempted.

Warwick and Berry have found that sheep eggs transferred to goats will develop into fetuses of 30- to 45-day gestational ages. Although goat eggs transplanted to sheep also implanted successfully, the embryos died at 22 days of gestation.

A line of approach currently being pursued that may lead to the successful transgression of species barriers by transferred blastocysts entails substitution of the inner cell mass in host-type blastocysts by inner cell masses from blastocysts of the alien donor species. Transfer of these chimeric or composite blastocysts and their subsequent development avoids direct confrontation of maternal uterine tissue by cells of an alien species.

The Peritrophoblastic Fibrinoid Hypothesis

On the basis of electron-microscopic and histochemical studies on mouse placentas, Kirby and his associates affirmed that the trophoblast represents an immunological buffer zone between mother and fetus and, like Bardawil and Toy, attributed the barrier properties to extracellular material. They suggested that transplantation (and presumably organ specific) antigens are present in trophoblast cells but are probably unable to escape or express themselves effectively because each trophoblast cell is surrounded by a layer of amorphous, electron-dense, fibrinoid material of mucopolysaccharide nature ranging from 0.1–2.0 μ in thickness. They drew attention to the close chemical similarity that exists between the intercellular matrix of the hamster's cheek pouch connective tissue (which appears to underlie the immunological privilege that this highly vascular organ normally extends to allografts and some xenografts) and the placental fibrinoid material. However, they omitted to stress one important difference between the two situations: whereas hamster cheek pouch is unable to afford any protection to vascularized allografts against an extant state of sensitivity, the fibrinoid associated with trophoblast cells apparently does have this property.

Sustaining the notion that peritrophoblastic fibrinoid material fulfills an immunologic masking role is the observation that its amount is related to the degree of immunogenetic disparity between mother and her fetus. Kirby and his associates claimed that histocompatible fetuses have less fibrinoid than F_1 fetuses or homozygous fetuses resulting from transfer of zygotes between females of different inbred strains.

Apart from trophoblast, the only other tissue whose cells can withstand transplantation immunity is cartilage. Studies on chondrocytes that have been isolated enzymically from their matrix indicate that these cells do express transplantation antigens and are fully susceptible to transplantation immunity. However, the avascularity and physicochemical properties of the matrix which these cells secrete and within which they are normally located not only prevents them from sensitizing their host but also affords them protection from the familiar hazards of transplantation immunity.

Evidence That Trophoblast Possesses "Masked" Alloantigens

Drs. Currie and Bagshawe have made observations suggestive of the association of transplantation antigens with trophoblast cells. When these cells were explanted *in vitro* with lymphocytes of maternal or alien donor origin, they underwent gross cytolysis, and postgestational choriocarcinoma cells underwent a similar fate when exposed to lymphocytes from the affected woman. That this *in vitro,* lymphocyte-trophoblastic cell interaction was immunologically specific was evidenced by the finding that trophoblastic cells confronted *in vitro* by lymphocytes of their *own* genetic constitution were not damaged.

What appears to be much more convincing evidence of the presence of transplantation antigens on mouse trophoblast cells and of their normal masking by pericellular layers of sialomucin was subsequently presented by these investigators. They found that treatment of ectoplacental cone cells from 7½-day old mouse embryos with neuraminidase *in vitro* enabled them to sensitize unrelated adult hosts against subsequent test skin allografts of their own genetic constitution. In view of the significance of this observation it is surprising that it has not yet received independent confirmation or has been extended to other strain combinations of mice or to other species. It is pertinent to state that neuraminidase, which specifically removes sialic acid groups from sialomucins, is capable of revealing normally covert antigenic determinants on certain types of tumor cells which secrete sialomucin. Such tumors can override appreciable histoincompatibility barriers. It has also been reported that treatment of mouse tumor cells with heparin or various sulfated mucopolysaccharides may lead to the "suppression" of certain isoantigens that are normally present, enabling the cells to survive allotransplantation.

Exactly how the peritrophoblastic layer of fibrinoid or sialomucin accomplishes its alleged immunologic quarantining effect is still the subject of speculation. Currie and Bagshawe suggested that by virtue of free carboxyl groups on sialic acid it confers a negative charge on the cell. Since lymphocytes likewise carry a negative charge, electrochemical repulsion *in vivo* prevents them from interacting with or attacking trophoblast cells. Subsequently Drs. Jones and Kemp have criticized this thesis as an oversimplification of the *modus operandi* of sialomucin in the "self-isolation" of fetal trophoblast. They believe that, irrespective of genetic differences between them, cells are probably held together by chemical bonds at adhesive sites on their surfaces. This probably accounts for the firm initial adhesion of the trophoblast cells to genetically different maternal endometrial cells during the early stages of development. Probably as a consequence of the fusion that occurs between trophoblast and maternal endometrial cells some kind of "informational" exchange takes place between these two cells types and trophoblast may be able to recognize its "genetic disaffinity" with the uterine epithelium and respond by secreting an intervening layer of sialomucin to which trophoblast and decidua probably contribute, thus quarantining itself. These authors further postulate that this material renders the outer surface of the trophoblast cells non-adhesive by masking the adhesive sites that had previously united tropho-blastic to uterine epithelial cells. Masking of these sites might also prevent maternal lymphocytes from establishing immunologically meaningful con-tactual relationships with trophoblast.

GROUNDS FOR CONCERN ABOUT IDENTIFICATION OF THE TROPHOBLAST-ASSOCIATED QUARANTINING BARRIER

Both the source of the trophoblast-associated sialomucin and its con-stancy of association with trophoblast in different species have yet to be placed on an experimental basis. There is conflicting evidence from two independent groups of investigators who employed electron microscopy, concerning the presence or absence of pericellular coatings of sialomucin on mouse trophoblast cells of blastocystic origin growing beneath the renal capsules of both syngeneic and allogeneic male hosts.

In a study of the rat placenta, Dr. John Martinek's findings indicated that at no time from mid-gestation to term does electron-dense fibrinoid material form an intact barrier between the fetal trophoblastic giant cells and maternal decidual cells, though increased amounts of interfacial fibri-noid were noted as the time of parturition approached. Throughout the latter half of pregnancy, significant amounts of viable trophoblast and decidual tissue appeared to be juxtaposed intimately. Martinek made similar observations in the mouse. In the rabbit placenta, prominent depositions of fibrinoid material have been reported to occur in the intercellular area of the trophoblastic cell layer but none of this material was demonstrable on trophoblastic villi.

Dr. Ralph Wynn's careful comparative ultrastructural studies of sev-eral different types of hemochorial placenta, including that of man, revealed material morphologically identical to the trophoblast cell-associated fibri-noid described by Kirby and his associates in the murine placenta. Wynn felt, however, that the fibrinoid he was studying was produced by the decidua. He discerned a positive correlation among invasiveness of the trophoblast, ultrastructural complexity of the decidua, the extent of necrosis of adjacent fetal and maternal tissues, and the formation of noncellular barriers. He regarded the demonstrable "fibrinoids" merely as *effects* of cellular interactions between trophoblast and endometrium rather than as factors playing a primary role in the immunologic protection of alien trophoblastic cells. In the epitheliochorial placentas of cows and sows, microvilli of chorionic and endometrial epithelia intermingle without sig-nificant necrosis and without deposition of fibrinoid. However, an extracel-lular coat of mucopolysaccharides closely resembling that associated with epithelial microvilli of other tissues, such as the intestinal mucosa that enjoys no exemption of rejection, was demonstrable. Of course, as Wynn points out, in simple placentas of this type, where the trophoblast is not normally exposed to immunologically competent maternal lymphocytes, there may be no need for either trophoblastic or extratrophoblastic protection.

It is obvious that much more solid evidence in its favor is required before Kirby's thesis that a trophoblast-associated sialomucin layer is the seat of the immunologic quarantining of the fetus can become generally accepted.

The Zona Pellucida

It has been suggested that the zona pellucida, which forms a protective coat around the embryo from fertilization almost to implantation and is impermeable to many proteins and to cells, may afford immunologic protection to fertilized eggs prior to the formation of the trophoblastic barrier in females who, for some reason, are hypersensitive to their mate's alien tissue antigens. The occasional survival of ectopically transplanted mouse eggs in hyperimmune hosts has been attributed to protection afforded by a persistent zona pellucida. Direct evidence that the zona can confer protection upon blastocysts against both cellular and humoral immunity has been forthcoming from *in vitro* studies.

Some doubt about the immunological significance of this membrane *in vivo* was cast by the results of one of Kirby's experiments, however. Using appropriate endocrinological procedures he deliberately prolonged the zona-free existence of H-2 locus-incompatible blastocysts in the uteri of hyperimmunized females. Despite their prolonged firm attachment to the wall of the host uterus in a zona-free state, there was no evidence that the survival rate of genetically susceptible zygotes differed significantly from that of control blastocysts. However, the quarantine afforded the zona-free blastocysts could have been secondary to the afferent blockade produced by the developing decidua.

REFERENCES

Beer, A. E., and Billingham, R. E. 1971. "Immunobiology of mammalian reproduction." *Adv. Immunol.* **14**:1–84.

Bratanov, K. 1969. "Antibodies in the reproductive process in the female." In *Immunology and reproduction* (R. G. Edwards, ed.). International Publications, New York, pp. 175–189.

Breyere, E. J., and Sprenger, W. W. 1969. "Evidence of allograft rejection of the conceptus." *Transpl. Proc.* **1**:71–75.

Chapman, V. M., Ansell, J. D., and McLaren, A. 1972. "Trophoblast giant cell differentiation in the mouse: Expression of glucose phosphate isomerase (GPI-1) electrophoretic variants in transferred and chimeric embryos." *Developmental Biol.* **29**:48–54.

Edidin, M. 1972. "Histocompatibility genes, transplantation antigens, and pregnancy." In *Transplantation antigens* (B. D. Kahan and R. A. Reisfeld, ed.). Academic Press, New York, pp. 75–114.

Heyner, S. 1973. "The antigenicity of cartilage grafts." *Surg., Gynecol., Obstet.* **136**:298–305.

Jackson, B. T. 1967. "Immunologic aspects of the fetus and fetal-maternal relationships." *Surgery* **62**:232–237.

Jones, B. M., and Kemp, R. B. 1969. "Self-isolation of the foetal trophoblast." *Nature* (London) **221**:829–831.

Kirby, D. R. S. 1968. "Transplantation and pregnancy," In *Human Transplantation* (F. T. Rapaport and J. Dausset, ed.). Grune and Stratton, New York, pp. 565–586.

Lanman, J. T. 1965. "Transplantation immunity in mammalian pregnancy: Mechanisms of fetal protection against immunologic rejection." *J. Pediat.* **66**:525–540.

Lanman, J. T., and Herod, L. 1965. "Homograft immunity in pregnancy. The placental transfer of cytotoxic antibody in rabbits." *J. Exp. Med.* **122**: 579–586.

Medawar, P. B. 1953. "Some immunological and endocrinological problems raised by the evolution of viviparity in vertebrates." *Symp. Soc. Exp. Biol.* **11**:320–338.

Palm, J., Heyner, S., and Brinster, R. L. 1971. "Differential immunofluorescence of fertilized mouse eggs with H-2 and non-H-2 antibody." *J. Exp. Med.* **133**:1282–1293.

Scott, J. R., Pitkin, R. M., and Chaudhuri, T. K. 1973. "The placenta: Immunologic or hemodynamic protector of the fetus?" *Am. J. Obstet. Gynecol* **117**:1109–1115.

Seigler, H. F., and Metzgar, R. S. 1972. "Transplantation antigens of the human fetus, trophoblast, and spermatozoa." In *Transplantation antigens* (B. D. Kahan and R. A. Reisfeld, ed.). Academic Press, New York, pp. 115–123.

Simmons, R. L., and Russell, P. S. 1962. "The antigenicity of mouse trophoblast." *Ann N.Y. Acad. Sci.* **99**:717–732.

Simmons, R. L., and Russell, P. S. 1966. "The histocompatibility antigens of fertilized mouse eggs and trophoblast." *Ann. N.Y. Acad. Sci.* **129**: 35–45.

Warwick, B. L., and Berry, R. O. 1949. "Intergeneric and intraspecific embryo transfer: In sheep and goats." *J. Hered.* **40**:297–393.

Wynn, R. M. 1967. "Fetomaternal cellular relations in human basal plate: An ultrastructural study of the placenta." *Am. J. Obstet. Gynecol.* **97**: 832–850.

Wynn, R. M. 1969. "Noncellular components of the placenta." *Am. J. Obstet. Gynecol.* **103**:723–739.

Chapter 7

Choriocarcinoma

From the immunological point of view no tumor presents a greater paradox than choriocarcinoma of gestational origin. It is a highly malignant, invasive derivative of the fetal trophoblastic epithelium that develops in the mother within a highly variable interval following a conception. The latter may have resulted in a hydatidiform mole—i.e., an abnormal vesicular mass of placental tissue, including trophoblast, from which the fetus may or may not have disappeared, an ectopic pregnancy, an abortion, or a perfectly normal birth. Choriocarcinomas metastasize very readily via the veins, involving many tissues and organs, especially the brain and lungs, in addition to the uterus and other pelvic organs. What is so remarkable about these tumors is that, despite their unquestionable *fetal* origin and therefore alien genetic status as grafts, they are nearly always fatal in untreated patients. It is important to mention, however, that these tumors do show a very definite complete, spontaneous regression rate that, although less than 5%, is nevertheless higher than that of any other kind of malignancy in man.

Choriocarcinoma is still the only malignant neoplasm that is curable even after metastatic dissemination has occurred. The remarkable degree of curability of choriocarcinoma with drugs, dating back to 1956, depends in part upon its susceptibility to folic acid antagonists, especially methotrexate. The progress of eradication of the malignant cells with cytotoxic drugs can readily be estimated by monitoring the patient's serum with a very sensitive radioimmunoassay procedure to detect the human chorionic gonadotropin (HCG) produced by them (see Fig. 7-1).

Apart from posing an immunologic problem, choriocarcinoma poses an epidemiologic one. It occurs 10 times more frequently among the native populations of the Middle East and Asia than in Caucasians. All the available evidence suggests that socioeconomic as well as genetic (see below) factors play an important role in this variable incidence of trophoblastic neoplasms. A final anomaly of choriocarcinoma is the absence, or extreme rarity, of homologues in other species (see below).

97

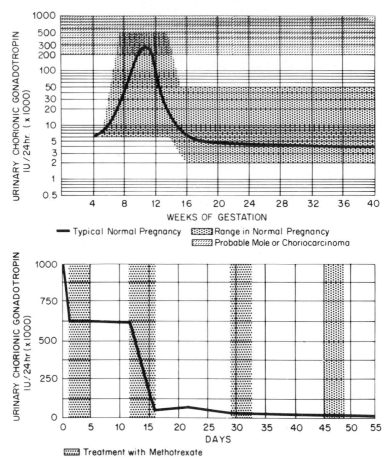

Fig. 7-1. In normal pregnancy, the chorionic gonadotropin titer reaches its peak between 8 and 12 weeks of pregnancy and then falls quite rapidly, as shown in this graph. Persistent elevation equal to or higher than the normal level is typical of trophoblastic disease.

It is interesting to note that with breast cancer, too, a significant disparity exists between the incidences among women in Caucasian and Oriental populations, but the trend is in the opposite direction to that seen with choriocarcinoma. The risk of a Caucasian resident of the United States developing mammary carcinoma in her lifetime (1 in 17), is five to six times greater than for an Oriental woman living in the Orient. Dr. Philip Cole has shown that both genetic and environmental (probably in part dietary) factors underlie this difference.

The Immunotherapeutic Approach

Cognizance of the alien genetic status of choriocarcinoma of gestational origin has prompted several groups of investigators to immunize affected women against their husbands' tissue antigens, by means of skin grafts and/or injections of viable peripheral blood leukocytes, in the hope of heightening their apparent ineffective resistance to the alien tumor cells bearing paternally inherited histocompatibility genes and presumably their products—i.e., transplantation antigens. This simple and very rational immunotherapeutic approach has usually been employed in cases where attempts to control the tumor by surgery and chemotherapy have failed. Unfortunately, no unequivocal successes have been reported and the patients have usually succumbed to their tumors despite the fact that they had developed a strong immunity to skin grafts from their husbands or, in one case, to a skin graft from a child syngeneic with her mother's tumor.

Most workers have noted that the intensity of the reactions of some of their patients to grafts of their husband's skin was markedly inferior to their reactions to concomitant grafts from unrelated donors or to the known response of healthy volunteers to skin grafts from unrelated donors. This observation has focused attention upon the possibility that exposure to the tumor, possibly in conjunction with chemotherapy, might have resulted in a specific impairment of the patient's capacity to react against the antigens concerned, as either a consequence of the induction of immunological tolerance or the development of "enhancing" or "blocking" isoantibodies. Evidence of the presence of antibodies reactive with their husbands' leukocytes in the sera of some patients has afforded some support for the latter premise. It seems most unlikely, however, that the tumor tissue alone was responsible for the formation of these antibodies, although it might have increased their titer.

Unfortunately, there are no appropriate control data available for these interesting skin grafting studies on choriocarcinoma patients in the sense that there is no information concerning the survival times of skin grafts from their husbands and from unrelated donors on *normal* women. As we shall see, in experimental animals, repeated matings and pregnancies by an urelated male can specifically weaken a female's reactivity to subsequent allografts of skin or other tissues from that male or from a genetically similar one (see page 127).

Evidence of Host Resistance

There are a number of clinical observations that uphold the general belief that patients can develop a weak immunity against choriocarcinomas of gestational origin: (1) When the aggregate tumor mass has been reduced to a low level by chemotherapy, often in conjunction with surgery, there may follow a long-term high remission that is much more impressive than that obtainable by treatment of any other kind of sarcoma or carcinoma. (2) Histological study of tumor specimens has revealed that leukocytic infiltration, in which lymphocytes participate, occurs in approximately 50% of the patients. More important, there seems to be a significant correlation between the intensity of this leukocytic response on the part of the host and the susceptibility of the tumor to chemotherapy. (3) There are well-documented instances of complete spontaneous remissions of choriocarcinoma and in some of these there was evidence of a host cellular response when surgically excised tumor material was examined.

We must not neglect the fact, however, that the normal precursor cells of this particular tumor, the cytotrophoblast cells, unlike precursors of practically all other types of tumor, have a finite life-span that barely exceeds the gestation period of the species concerned. Thus regression of some choriocarcinomas might simply reflect the eventual operation of this principle.

In contradistinction to the allogeneic choriocarcinomas of gestational origin, there are also autochthonous choriocarcinomas that originate in the gonads of both males and females. Whereas spread of the gestational form of the tumor by lymphatic routes and its presence in regional lymph nodes is rare, this is not the case with the autochthonous tumors, hinting at the operation of immunologic resistance in the case of the former. Although exceptions exist, the results of chemotherapeutic treatment of patients with primary ovarian or testicular choriocarcinomas are markedly inferior to those obtainable in patients with the allogeneic (gestational) form of the tumor. As Dr. K. D. Bagshawe of Fulham Hospital, London, has pointed out, however, in the light of the probability that the tumors of gonadal origin probably include malignant cell lineages of other types, which are less susceptible to chemotherapy, this observation loses some of its immunological significance.

The fact that women with gestational choriocarcinoma respond better to chemotherapy initiated soon after the onset of the disease hints that feebly antigenic tumors that are allowed to persist are capable of inducing tolerance or enhancement in their hosts, just as weakly immunogenic allografts of normal tissues, as well as kidney and cardiac transplants, are able to do in experimental animals.

ANTIGENIC CHARACTER OF THE TROPHOBLAST

If the spontaneous regression of choriocarcinomas in untreated patients and the cures obtainable by chemotherapy do reflect the operation of host immunologic resistance or surveillance processes, there are several kinds of antigenic determinants against which these responses may be directed:

1. A tumor-specific antigen, behaving like a weak cellular transplantation antigen, absent from normal trophoblast, and of the type that characterizes many kinds of tumor. Presently, the evidence for the existence of such an antigen is rather weak.

2. A cytospecific or organ-specific antigen(s) that choriocarcinoma may share with normal trophoblast, analogous to the organ-specific antigens associated with thyroid, brain, and testis. Evidence that a unique antigenic determinant is probably associated with trophoblast will shortly be considered in Chapter 6. In this regard, human chorionic gonadotropin (HCG) and human placental lactogen (or somatomammotropin) (HPL) are hormones synthesized by the trophoblast that may confer autoantigenicity upon the cells that secrete them.

3. Blood group antigens, especially those of the ABO system, that are important as transplantation antigens in organ transplantation.

4. Human leukocyte antigens (HL-A antigens) serologically most readily detectable on leukocytes but also present on many different cell types. Some of these play an important role in determining histocompatibility.

It has been suggested that a predisposing factor in the progressive development of choriocarcinoma may be the absence of a maternal immune response to normal trophoblast that has the unique, functionally important property of invading host tissue in a vigorous, cancer-like manner in the process of placental formation. The nature of the normal process responsible for limiting this benign invasion is still open to speculation. The fact that trophoblastic invasion is not overtly more extensive in isogenic strains of animals than in outbred animals rules out segregating alloantigens as the basis of the control (see Chapter 1). The possibility remains, however, that fetal-maternal differences with respect to blood group and other antigens might have some influence on the invasive, proliferative, and survival potential of choriocarcinomas of gestational origin.

FETAL-MATERNAL ALLOANTIGENIC COMPATIBILITY AS A PREDISPOSING FACTOR

Consanguineous marriages, which are said to be relatively frequent in some geographic areas where the tumor incidence is high, have been suggested as a predisposing factor in the development of choriocarcinoma. This view is colored by a report that both wives of a local prince, one his first cousin and the other his second cousin, developed choriocarcinoma within a month of each other.

Comparison of the ABO and HL-A antigens of patients with those of their tumors should, in theory, afford a means of determining whether compatibility of the offending fetus with respect to these important histocompatibility systems is an important predisposing factor for the development of choriocarcinoma. Unfortunately, neither of these series of determinants is currently detectable on trophoblastic tumor cells so that an indirect approach had to be adopted. Essentially, this involves deducing the probable tissue types of the offending conceptus from typing data on the affected woman, her husband, and other members of the family. Of course, in those instances where the offending pregnancy resulted in a healthy infant, blood and tissue typing provides the necessary information about the tumor directly. Dr. Bagshawe and his associates in London have studied a series of 24 families in which the patient, husband, and child from whose trophoblast the tumor originated were available. Their findings make it perfectly clear that gestational choriocarcinoma can occur despite incompatibility with regard to both ABO and HL-A antigens, utterly refuting the notion that a *necessary* condition for the development of these tumors is immunogenetic compatibility of the fetus with its mother. Moreover, in some instances, it has been shown that the tumor continued to flourish in the face of HL-A antibodies in the patient's serum directed against the antigens of the child (which are probably present in some form on the tumor cells). Here initiation of the immunization must be attributed to pregnancy though the antibody titers may, in some instances, have been boosted by blood transfusion and possibly by antigenic material of tumor origin. Since antibodies were present in patients who succumbed to their disease as well as in those in whom treatment was successful no prognostic significance can be attached to their presence. Recently Drs. Lawler, Klouda, and Bagshawe have shown that "first-pregnancy" hydatiform molar tissue, devoid of all other fetal tissue elements including blood, can evoke HL-A antibodies in affected females. This is further evidence that HL-A antigens are associated with trophoblastic tissue.

The probability of a woman developing choriocarcinoma associated with a pregnancy appears to be determined in part by her own ABO blood group and in part by that of her husband. Early suggestive evidence that women of group A have a greater chance of developing choriocarcinoma than those of group O has been substantiated and shown to depend also on the blood groups of their husbands. For example, a group A woman married to a group O male is 10 times more likely to develop the tumor than if she'd picked a group A spouse, and group AB patients with choriocarcinoma often show rapid progression of their tumors. Clinically, group A patients tend to have rapidly progressive tumors that do not respond well to chemotherapy and group A females married to group A males are at lowest risk.

Although these interesting observations show very clearly that genetic factors in both mother and conceptus exert an important influence on the development of choriocarcinoma, they are not explicable in terms of a simple, immunogenetic hypothesis. Certainly women of blood groups A, AB, and B are more likely to have conceptuses that do not confront them with alien antigens of this group than group O women. This could explain the decreased risk that women of this latter type have of developing the tumor. What is difficult to account for is the excess risk associated with A♀ × O♂ matings as compared with A♀ × A♂ matings since both can only produce conceptuses that are compatible with the mothers with regard to these antigens.

HL-A ANTIGENS AND CHORIOCARCINOMA

Several investigations have been made of the HL-A antigens of women with gestational choriocarcinoma, their husbands, and children. In a growing number of cases availability of the actual child who "donated" the malignant allograft to its mother has enabled the antigenic disparity between tumor and mother to be established with a high degree of certainty. The results indicate that only a small proportion of patients do in fact have HL-A compatible tumors—i.e., those that could not confront them with one or more alien HL-A specificities. The data do hint, however, that a slightly increased risk of a tumor developing is associated with feto-maternal histocompatibility at this locus. Nevertheless, the fact that chemotherapy is usually successful even in the presence of proved or very probable histocompatibility indicates that HL-A incompatibility is not a prerequisite to obtain cures with chemotherapy, though the prognosis in general seems to be poorer when compatibility prevails.

Consistent with these rather tentative, provisional conclusions are the findings from a recent survey of Greenland Eskimos among whom the incidence of choriocarcinoma is relatively high, like that of Southeast Asian populations. Some HL-A antigens among Eskimos are much more frequent than among Caucasians (for example, 81% are HL-A 9 positive, as compared with 20% in Caucasians). As a consequence of this situation a much higher proportion of Eskimo conceptuses are compatible with their mothers at this locus.

Finally, when the results of studies on the ABO and HL-A antigens are compared, it appears that the influence of the former is greater than that of the latter in determining the risk of a given fetal-maternal situation giving rise to choriocarcinoma.

Three important unresolved questions about choriocarcinoma are

1. Unlike other tumors that have been tested, would grafts of this

tumor thrive in a high proportion of normal volunteer hosts genetically unrelated to the donors? Because of the obvious risk involved in performing the test, we shall never be able to answer this question so far as man is concerned.

2. Why is it that when a pregnancy results in a normal birth as well as choriocarcinoma in the mother, the infant is only very rarely affected by this malignant derivative of its *own* placenta?

3. What is a normal multiparous woman's reactivity to tissue allografts from her husband? Repeatedly exposed to his alien tissue antigens via her reproductive tract through sexual intercourse and pregnancies, her initial virginal immunological reactivity may well have undergone specific weakening through the induction of tolerance and/or immunologic enhancement. This might explain the observed apparent diminished reactivity of patients to skin grafts from their husbands, but not from unrelated donors.

Another important empirical finding to be taken into consideration in this context is that orthotopic skin allografts, in experimental animals, are much more exacting in their genetic requirements for survival than allografts of other tissues and organs. For example, in rats, heart and renal transplants can override degrees of histoincompatibility sufficient to procure prompt rejection of skin allografts. An orthotopic skin graft is thus an exacting "control" with which to compare these naturally occurring malignant allotransplants—choriocarcinomas.

Further, large-scale sophisticated blood- and tissue-typing studies on patients with gestational choriocarcinoma and their families, among both high- and low-incidence populations, will probably enlighten us concerning the basis of the marked geographical variations that exist, the prognosis for given cases, and possibly the etiology.

We must not neglect the fact that blood groups and HL-A types represent variations in the fine chemical structure of cell surface components that are detectable by virtue of their ability to elicit isoimmune reactions. It does not necessarily follow that all phenomena or diseases that have a statistically significant association with particular isoantigens have an immunologically based etiology. For example, group O individuals are about 40% more likely to develop duodenal ulcers than group A, B, or AB subjects, and nonsecretors of blood group substances are about 50% more liable to develop ulcers than secretors. Clearly it would be difficult to account for this situation on an immunological basis. The explanation of these disparities seems to turn in part upon group O individuals possessing a larger gastric secretory cell mass. In the case of choriocarcinoma, phenotypic variations with regard to trophoblast cell antigens might affect the penetrability to a venereally or otherwise transmitted viral agent. Although these agents have been sought by ultrastructural analysis of both hydatiform moles and choriocarcinomas, they have never been unequivocally demonstrated.

Propagability of Choriocarcinoma in Hamsters

Dr. Roy Hertz has established the serial propagability of gestational choriocarcinomas from seven patients in the cheek pouches of both normal and cortisone-treated or antilymphocyte serum-treated (i.e., immunosuppressed) Syrian hamsters. The transplanted tumor tissue usually attains its maximal size within about 15 days after which it is overcome by the host's immunologic response, so that by 30 days only a small residual scar remains. That the cells of these propagated tumors have retained their original structure and function has been attested by light and electron microscopy, as well as hormonal determinations. Nevertheless, they have consistently failed to metastasize in the hamster hosts. Since these animal-propagated tumors do retain their susceptibility to methotrexate and other drugs, they afford potentially useful models for screening other chemotherapeutic agents.

Choriocarcinoma in Other Species

There are few reports of the occurrence of choriocarcinoma in other species. Additional examples are one case in the nine-banded armadillo, one possible case in a cow, and one in a rhesus monkey. Shintani has claimed considerable success, however, in the chemical induction of these tumors in rats. He fetectomizes pregnant females on the ninth through tenth day of pregnancy and then implants pellets of beeswax containing 9,10-dimethyl,1,2-benzanthracene into the embryonic sacs. A small proportion of the tumors that developed were identified as choriocarcinomas on the basis of both gross and microscopic appearance. Some of these tumors metastasized to the lungs. The induction of similar tumors in rats of an inbred strain would facilitate analysis of the ability of these tumors to grow in both normal and specifically presensitized allogeneic hosts. No explanation can be offered for the apparent almost complete restriction of choriocarcinoma to humans unless, following Dr. William Ober, one is prepared to attach some significance to the empiric fact that, unlike females of all other species, human females have abandoned the habit of eating their placentas after giving birth.

A Transmissible Venereal Tumor in the Dog

With the exception of leukocytes that may be transmitted via the milk (see Chapter 14) the only other instance known to us of the natural, successful transplantation of allogeneic cells is a transmissible venereal lymphosarcoma of the dog. The majority of these tumors arise on or in close proximity to the external genitalia and are transmitted by coition. The first known experimental transmission of a tumor, performed by Novinski in 1876, employed this particular neoplasm and established its experimental propagability in dogs. Metastases are infrequent and only rarely are these tumors fatal. They normally attain a considerable size over a several-month period and then regress and disappear. Following spontaneous regression, dogs are refractory to further transplantation of the tumor. Partial surgical removal of these tumors usually incites complete regression and a resistant state in the host.

The results of cytogenetic studies sustain the thesis that this is a tumor of *unitary* origin that has subsequently maintained itself in the species through the survival and proliferation of transmitted malignant cells in allogeneic hosts rather than through the transformation of host cells by a viral agent. So far no one has determined how these tumor cells manage to overcome histocompatibility barriers so successfully. Impressed by the intriguing theoretical problems posed by this tumor the late Dr. P. A. Gorer suggested in 1960 that "were it not for the antigenic diversity of most species and the existence of a mechanism to react against the antigens, contagious tumors would be relatively common."

REFERENCES

Bagshawe, K. D. 1969. *Choriocarcinoma*. Williams and Wilkins, Baltimore.

Bagshawe, K. D., Rawlins, G., Pike, M. C., and Lawler, S. 1971. "ABO blood groups in trophoblastic neoplasia." *Lancet*. i:553–557.

Cole, P. 1974. "Epidemiology of human breast cancer." *J. Invest. Dermatol.* 63:133–137.

Hagegawa, T. 1971. *Trophoblastic neoplasia*. Williams and Wilkins, Baltimore.

Holland, J. F., and Hreshchyshyn, M. M., ed. 1967. *Choriocarcinoma*. Vol. 3. UICC Monograph Series. Springer-Verlag, New York.

Kissmeyer-Nielsen, F., and Thorsby, E. 1970. "Human transplantation antigens." *Transpl. Rev.* 4:1–176.

Lewis, J. L., and Terasaki, P. I. 1971. "HL-A leukocyte antigen studies in women with gestational trophoblastic neoplasm." *Am. J. Obstet. Gynecol.* 111:547–552.

Park, W. W. 1971. *Choriocarcinoma. A study of its pathology*. F. A. Davis, Philadelphia.

Smith, H. A., Jones, T. C., and Hunt, R. D. 1972. *Veterinary pathology*. Lea and Febiger, Philadelphia (for information about the transmissible venereal tumors in dogs).

Walford, R. L., Smith, G. S., and Walters, H. 1971. "Histocompatibility systems and disease states with particular reference to cancer." *Transpl. Rev.* **7**:78–111.

Chapter 8

Organ-Specific Antigens of the Placenta

Previously we have considered the extent to which the placenta or, more specifically, its syncytial trophoblast as well as choriocarcinoma express antigens determined by segregating histocompatibility genes. The question to which we shall address ourselves in this chapter is whether this transitory organ possesses antigens that are unique unto itself, i.e., *organ-specific* antigens, and with what structural components are they associated.

Trophoblast is a highly specialized tissue with unique ultrastructural features and no doubt with distinctive ingredients and products that in man include chorionic gonadotropin and chorionic somatomammotropin as well as cells whose DNA content is far greater than that of any other nucleate cells. In addition it appears to have "immunologic self-quarantining" properties, analogous to those associated with the testis and the brain. Apart from a possible transient exposure to their own trophoblast during fetal life, males never become reexposed to it through pregnancy, as adults. In the light of these considerations there is a *prima facie* case that this tissue, like testis, brain and lens, may contain its own "private" autoantigens of which the mature animal has never become tolerant and consequently against which it might be able to react immunologically. If an individual did become tolerant of her own placental antigens during fetal life, the likelihood is that, through absence of the necessary "tolerance"-maintaining antigenic stimulus from parturition onward the unresponsive state would disappear.

Interest in the possible organ-specific antigenicity of the placenta was stimulated at the beginning of the century by the suggestion that the clinically important toxemias of pregnancy might, in some way, be the result of maternal sensitization against undefined placental antigens, secondarily leading to renal damage and central nervous system involvement.

Biological Activity of Heterologous Antiplacental Serum

The principle that an antiserum raised in a member of one species against placental homogenates, etc., from a member of another species is capable of interrupting pregnancies in the species that provided the antigen was first established in guinea pigs and rabbits by Dobrowolski in 1903. Subsequent investigators have shown that placental degeneration and fetal death can be procured by the administration of heterologous antiplacental serum to mice, rats, and rhesus monkeys and that antibodies to erythrocytes contaminating the placental homogenates used as antigen were not responsible for this effect. These observations suggested the existence of a specific antigen(s) in placental tissue.

Of particular importance from the clinical viewpoint were reports that these antiplacental sera also had a powerful nephrotoxic effect. In neither rats nor dogs, however, have heterologous antikidney sera of proved nephrotoxic potency been found to damage placentas. It is interesting to note though that Brent and Averich found that administration of nephrotoxic serum to rats on the ninth day of gestation caused the development of fetal congenital abnormalities. This might have resulted from anoxia associated with damage to the placenta.

Cross-Reactivity Between Renal and Placental Antigens

Elucidation of the nature and distribution of the antigens that kidney and placenta appear to share in common has been the objective of many studies using either crude tissue homogenates or definable fractions prepared therefrom by differential centrifugation and other means. Administration of the antigenic material in CFA is virtually essential to stimulate antibody formation. After appropriate absorptions with various types of cell or tissue homogenate the specificity of the antisera has been evaluated by *in vivo* organ toxicity tests, immunodiffusion, hemagglutination, application of direct or indirect fluorescent antibody procedures to freshly prepared sections of various tissues, and localization of passively administered antibodies *in vivo* by indirect fluorescent antibody or radioactively labeled antibody.

The results of these studies, which have been conducted in a variety of species including man, are fairly consistent and can be summarized as follows: (1) Antiplacental and renal antiglomerular basement membrane antibodies localize *in vitro* in a similar manner in the basement membranes of glomeruli, tubules, intertubular capillaries, and certain extracellular sites in the media and adventitia of arteries. (2) Both types of antisera display similar patterns of localization in placental tissue, on the basement membranes of the labyrinth and trophoblast, Reichert's membrane, and the yolk sac. (3) Soluble antigens common to placenta and kidney are demonstrable by immunodiffusion but cannot be localized immunohistologically. (4) Common or shared antigens are demonstrable in the mitochondrial and microsomal fractions of the placental trophoblast and renal proximal tubule epithelium (there is good evidence that the principal, if not the only, source of these antigens in the placenta is the trophoblast). (5) On the basis of results obtained with immunodiffusion and other studies, a *mixture* of antibodies is involved, indicating that kidney and placenta must share more than one antigen in common.

Attempts have been made to detect antibodies to placental tissue in the blood of pregnant women and there is one report of a circulating antibody to a placental polysaccharide. Postulating that if such antibodies are formed, they might easily be absorbed by trophoblastic tissue in the placenta, Dr. J. Hulka and his associates tested postpartum serum in both normal and toxemic pregnancies. They obtained evidence of specific binding of fluorescein-tagged maternal globulin by the syncytiothrophoblast, which they interpreted as indicative of the presence of antitrophoblast antibodies. These "antibodies" were detectable earlier in the latter part of pregnancy or postpartum period in women with toxemia than in normal pregnant women.

THE EXISTENCE OF A "PRIVATE" TISSUE-SPECIFIC ANTIGEN IN TROPHOBLAST

The findings of two entirely separate lines of investigation, with biological end points: (1) studies on the abortifacient property of antitrophoblast sera and (2) analysis of the growth of consecutive heterotopic grafts of trophoblast derived from blastocysts or ectoplacental cones in mice attest to the existence of a trophoblast-specific antigen(s).

Dr. Zeev Koren and his associates raised an antiserum in rabbits by inoculating them with homogenates of whole mouse placentas or relatively pure preparations of trophoblast cells incorporated in CFA. When aliquots of 0.25–0.5 ml of antiserum were injected intravenously into pregnant mice, on three separate occasions, pregnancy was consistently interrupted. Histological studies revealed focal areas of hemorrhage and necrosis in the placentas, as well as significant lesions in their livers and kidneys, suggestive of an immunologically induced glomerular nephritis in the latter organ. The use of an indirect fluorescent antibody technique to determine the fate of the passively transferred antitrophoblast antibody *in vivo* indicated a high degree of localization in trophoblast cells. Because of the complexity of the material used as antigen to immunize the rabbits and the fact that no absorptions were carried out, however, these interesting findings do not constitute decisive evidence that a specific antitrophoblast antibody (not present in antikidney serum) was responsible for aborting the mice.

Beer and associates, in an attempt further to clarify the autoantigenic status of the trophoblast, prepared antiserum by inoculating adult male rabbits with relatively pure preparations of viable trophoblast cells prepared from Fischer rat placentas of 12–14 days' gestation (see Fig. 8-1). The antigen was incorporated in CFA and inoculated into the foot pads on the initial occasion. Booster injections of viable suspensions of trophoblast cells were administered intravenously 3 and 4 weeks later. This protocol is essentially that which has proved satisfactory in raising biologically active antilymphocyte serum (ALS). Hemagglutinins were absorbed with rat erythrocytes. When this antiserum was administered intramuscularly to pregnant Fischer rats at a dosage level of 3 ml distributed over a 3-day period, it aborted them all, and also caused the deaths of 12% of them. Prior absorption of the antiserum with rat lymphoid cells, following absorption with erythrocytes, left its abortifacient property intact but rendered it totally harmless so far as the pregnant animals themselves were concerned.

Additional observations supporting the premise that an antibody specifically reactive with a distinctive component of trophoblast, rather than with an antigenic determinant shared in common with a variety of cell types, was responsible for the abortifacient property of the antitrophoblast serum include the following: (1) Neither rabbit antirat epidermal cell serum nor an antiserum raised against cells of fetuses *per se* harmed either pregnant rats or their fetuses. (2) The abortifacient activity of the erythrocyte and lymphocyte-absorbed antitrophoblast serum could be completely removed by absorption with suspensions of trophoblast cells. (3) The antiserum was effective in aborting rats of *any* strain. (4) Histological examination of the placentas of recipients of antitrophoblast serum revealed areas of hemorrhage and necrosis as well as infiltration of these organs by plasma cells, small lymphocytes, and polymorphonuclear leukocytes. The fetuses were edematous and macerated. Neither grossly nor microscopically were any lesions demonstrable in the mothers, however, indicating a high degree of tissue specificity. The finding that an antiserum raised against uterine decidual cells was devoid of abortifacient activity refuted the possibility that an antidecidual or an antiendometrial cell antibody was responsible for the biological activity of the antitrophoblast serum.

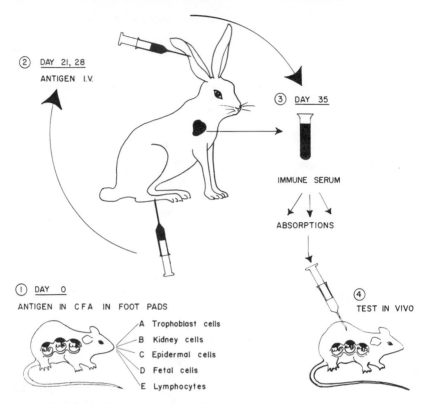

Fig. 8-1. Design of experiment that indicated the autoantigenic status of trophoblast cells. Suspensions of various types of tissue cells (A–E) were prepared in Hanks' solution from Fischer rats or their 18-day-old fetuses, mixed with Freund's adjuvant and injected into the hind foot pads of rabbits. Booster injections of cells in Hanks' solution were given intravenously on days 21 and 28. The animals were exsanguinated on day 35 and serum prepared. This was heat inactivated to remove complement and absorbed with Fischer erythrocytes to remove all red blood cell agglutinins. Aliquots of the various antisera were injected intramuscularly into pregnant rats to evaluate their abortifacient activity. Antitrophoblast serum, absorbed with lymphocytes was without toxicity for the pregnant rats and retained its abortifacient activity. This activity was completely removed by absorption with viable trophoblast cell suspensions. The other antisera tested had no abortifacient activity.

Experiments were also conducted to determine whether rats could be made to react against their *own* trophoblastic antigens. In one series of experiments, male Fischer rats were subjected to the standard immunization protocol, which was successful in the rabbit. Allogeneic DA strain trophoblast cells were used as antigen in the hope that the association of alien transplantation antigens with the putative, trophoblast-specific antigen might have an adjuvant effect. Antiserum harvested from these animals failed to prejudice pregnancy in Fischer rats. In a second series of experiments an unsuccessful attempt was made actively to sensitize Fischer females against subsequent pregnancies.

Finally it may be mentioned that as little as 1 ml of rabbit antirat trophoblast serum administered on a single occasion was effective in terminating pregnancy. Fetuses were equally susceptible to this antibody over the range 7–18 days postconception, and the antibody was found to be highly species-specific, having no activity in mice or hamsters.

In rhesus monkeys, too, Drs. Behrman and Amano of the University of Michigan have shown that pregnancy of 40–55 days duration can be terminated by intravenous injection of heterologous goat or rabbit anti-placental globulin. The latter was produced in response to inoculations of crude homogenates of monkey placentas in CFA. Abortion took place within 2–7 days of the injection of the monkeys with antiserum and no harm was caused to the mothers.

In this and other recent studies, immunodiffusion and immunoelectro-phoretic analyses of placental extracts have indicated the existence of at least one placental-specific antibody. The results of cytotoxic tests, using cultured monkey trophoblast cells as "targets," suggested a correlation between the antibody titers and the abortifacient properties of a given antiserum.

Bagshawe's observation that high dilutions of rabbit antisera raised against highly purified human chorionic gonadotropin were rapidly lethal to choriocarcinoma and normal trophoblast cells in vitro raised the inter-esting possibility that at least one antigen associated with trophoblast might prove to be a hormone or its receptor on the cell surface. A recent report from Tokyo, by Dr. Morisada and his associates, substantiates this inter-esting observation. These workers cultured human trophoblast from early pregnancies in cell-impermeable Millipore diffusion chambers inserted into the peritoneal cavities of rabbits. Prior immunization of the hosts with human chorionic gonadotropin resulted in selective damage to the syncytial layers of trophoblast, now believed to be the source of this hor-mone, after a week of culture; the cytotrophoblast manifested lesser de-grees of degeneration.

The second line of evidence in support of the existence of trophoblast-specific antigens derives from more or less concomitant but independent studies by Hulka and Mohr in the United States and Kirby in England. Hulka and Mohr compared the results of transplanting primary and sec-ondary grafts of ectoplacental cone tissue, prepared from C3H mouse embryos, beneath the renal capsules of male C57BL/6 host mice. Prior exposure of the hosts to a single intrarenal allograft of trophoblastic tissue reduced the incidence of successful secondary grafts and inhibited their growth. Lymphocytic infiltration was observed in association with both primary and secondary grafts, being slightly more intense in the latter. The authors interpreted their findings as indicative of sensitization of the hosts to trophoblast antigens, though the data afforded no clue as to their nature.

In a more recent study Hulka and co-workers succeeded in transferring the resistance elicited by primary intrarenal trophoblast allografts in mice to secondary syngeneic hosts by means of relatively low doses of spleen cells. Various control experiments indicated that the transferred resistance to trophoblast grafts was strain-specific, implying that histocompatibility antigens rather than an organ-specific antigens were involved.

Kirby reported that repeated transfer of quartets of C3H blastocysts, first beneath the renal capsules and later into the testes of C57BL/6 male hosts, resulted in a progressive diminution and, in some cases, the total inhibition of the ability of the blastocyst grafts to develop as evidenced by the decreased size of the hemorrhagic swellings (due to trophoblastic invasion) at the implantation sites. On the reasonable assumption that the phenomenon under study was immunologically based, conclusive evidence was obtained that the antigens responsible were *not* determined by histocompatibility genes but were probably tissue-specific. For example, when a single syngeneic blastocyst was transplanted to the testis of each of a group of C57 males, which had previously received four sets of C3H blastocysts, it grew with a significantly diminished vigor. Similar findings were obtained when the reciprocal experiment was performed; i.e., C57 blastocysts were transplanted to C3H male hosts.

In contrast to the inhibition of trophoblastic growth caused by repeated exposure of host mice to allogeneic blastocysts, when the hosts were finally challenged with skin allografts of the same genetic origin as the prior blastocyst grafts, their capacity to reject them was found to have been weakened as evidenced by prolongation of the skin graft survival.

Kirby also noted a progressive diminution in the size of the hemorrhagic lesions that developed at the implantation sites when consecutive sets of C3H blastocysts were transplanted to *syngeneic,* i.e., C3H hosts. This observation lends considerable support to the view that tissue-specific antigens are indeed associated with the trophoblast. In appraising the significance of these interesting findings, however, the possibility must be considered that the organ-specific antigens that seem to have been demonstrated may only be expressed by trophoblast at an early stage in its development—they may not be demonstrable in older placentas. Furthermore, to evaluate the possible biological significance of progressively attenuated growth of successive ectopically transplanted blastocysts it is necessary to study the development of ectopic blastocysts in multiparous mice—i.e., animals that have been repeatedly exposed to putative trophoblast-specific antigens as a consequence of normal pregnancies.

PARTURITION AS AN IMMUNOLOGICALLY
MEDIATED PROCESS

Parturition certainly represents an active repudiation of the fetoplacental unit by the mother and the suggestion was tentatively made by Dr. Lewis Thomas that degenerative changes occurring in the placenta as gestation proceeds might be caused by sensitization of the mother to a special organ-specific antigen that may be expressed relatively late in the maturation of this tissue. As Thomas was careful to point out, the consistent occurrence of parturition in inbred strains of rodents virtually precludes the possible involvement of transplantation antigens in such a mechanism. Two obvious implications of Thomas' premise are (1) Each of a series of pregnancies in a given female should be of somewhat shorter duration than its predecessor because of maternal sensitization to the antigens involved. (2) At least initial pregnancies should be of abnormally long duration in patients suffering from immunologic deficiency diseases or under chronic immunosuppressive therapy, such as recipients of renal allografts. As far as we are aware, there is no clinical evidence to sustain these predictions.

The late Dr. Albert Tyler suggested that parturition might be mediated by a graft-versus-host type of reactivity in which transplantation antigens are involved. Making the reasonable assumption that fetuses do not express all the transplantation antigens corresponding to their genotype during intrauterine life, and in the light of knowledge that fetuses can react against some transplantation antigens before birth, he postulated that even in the case of intrastrain pregnancies it might be possible for fetuses to "reject" their mothers. The remarkable constancy of the gestation period in many species, particularly in laboratory rodents, and the normal delivery at "expected" term of infants suffering from a variety of immunological deficiency diseases (including athymic or "nude" mice) known to prelude or impair their engaging in reactivity against allografts, makes this hypothesis virtually untenable.

Most of the available evidence indicates that it is the fetus rather than the mother who determines when gestation is to terminate with the onset of labor—i.e., uterine contractions leading to expulsion of the fetus and its sustaining placenta—and that the mechanisms involved are hormone-mediated.

TOXEMIA OF PREGNANCY

The disease known as toxemia of pregnancy—characterized by hypertension, edema, proteinuria, and occasionally convulsions—is a common complication of gestation, occurring in about 6% of all women late in their first pregnancy and responsible for about a third of maternal deaths in the United States per year. As a cause of perinatal death this condition is even more important. According to Drs. Hellman and Pritchard, "the cause of the toxemias of pregnancy, despite decades of intensive research, remains the great enigma of obstetrics and constitutes one of the most important unsolved problems in the whole field of human reproduction."

Since some authorities have implicated placental antigenicity as being causally responsible for this condition, critical examination of this concept falls within the scope of this book.

The following observations support, or have been cited as supporting, the premise that antigenicity of the placenta, probably its trophoblast, is in some way responsible for the disease.

1. There is cross-reactivity between antigens of placenta and kidney, and possibly those of the brain. The injection of some heterologous anti-placental sera may cause toxemia-like symptoms in experimental animals.

2. In women the symptoms normally disappear quite promptly following removal of the placenta by delivery of the fetus—the only effective treatment for the several forms of the disease.

3. Pathologic changes in the arterioles in the vascular bed of the placenta in patients with toxemia resemble those seen in the vasculature of an organ allograft undergoing rejection.

4. There is some evidence that placental size, and therefore possibly antigenic dose, is greater in women destined to develop toxemia. This might be indicative of increased trophoblastic invasion and possibly of impairment of homeostatic control mechanisms (possibly of an immunologic nature) that normally limit this process.

5. Statistical studies suggest that pregnancies resulting in toxemias tend to involve fetuses that are relatively histoincompatible with their mothers and the sex ratio of infants born of toxemic mothers is shifted toward a predominance of males.

6. The disease is primarily a disease of young women pregnant for the first time and does not commonly repeat itself in the second pregnancy by the same male even when the first pregnancy was very short and ended in an abortion. This finding is consistent with the possibility that in normal pregnancies "blocking" antibodies of some type are responsible for preventing the development of this condition.

7. The disease also occurs fairly frequently in association with hydatidiform mole and, again, rapid recovery follows the removal of this trophoblastic neoplasm, despite retention of some endocrinologically active trophoblast.

8. The incidence of the disease is much higher in lower socioeconomic groups where nutritional inadequacies and the absence of prenatal care are

common. In such populations there is evidence of a high incidence of deranged B lymphocyte function.

Findings that are not easily reconcilable with an immunological interpretation of toxemia are (1) In experimental contexts it is not easy to elicit either isoimmune or autoimmune responses to trophoblast even when adjuvants are used. (2) If trophoblastic antigens are involved, one would have expected to find the disease in patients with choriocarcinoma, however, it is rarely encountered, if at all, in such patients. (3) No antigen-antibody complexes have been found in association with the renal lesions of toxemia. (4) There is no evidence of an increased incidence of ABO or Rh blood group incompatibility or of postpartum leukocyte antibodies in toxemia patients.

REFERENCES

Beer, A. E., Billingham, R. E., and Yang, S. L. 1972. "Further evidence concerning the autoantigenic status of the trophoblast." *J. Exp. Med.* **135**: 1177–1184.

Behrman, S. J., and Amano, Y. 1972. "Monkey antiplacental serum as an abortifacient." *Contraception* **5**:357–368.

Bevans, M., Seegal, B. C., and Kaplan, R. 1955. "Glomerulonephritis produced in dogs by specific antisera. II. Pathological consequences following injection of rabbit antidog-placenta serum or antidog-kidney serum." *J. Exp. Med.* **102**:807–822.

Boss, J. H. 1965. "Antigenic relationships between placenta and kidney in humans." *Am. J. Obstet. Gynecol.* **93**:574–582.

Curzen, P. 1968. "The antigenicity of human placenta." *J. Obstet. Gynaecol. Brit. Com.* **75**:1128–1133.

Hellman, L. M., and Pritchard, J. A. 1970. *Williams' Obstetrics.* 14th ed., Appleton-Century-Croft, New York.

Hulka, J. F., and Mohr, K. 1968. "Trophoblast antigenicity demonstrated by altered challenge graft survival." *Science* **161**:696–698.

Kirby, D. R. S. 1968. "The immunologic consequences of extrauterine development of allogeneic mouse blastocysts." *Transplantation* **6**:1005–1009.

Kometani, K., and Behrman, S. J. 1971. The time of onset of placenta susceptibility in mice to heterologous anti-mouse placental serum." *Int. J. Fertil.* **16**:139–143.

Koren, Z., Abrams, G., and Behrman, S. J. 1968. "Antigenicity of mouse placental tissue." *Am. J. Obstet. Gynecol.* **102**:340–346.

Morisada, M., Yamaguchi, H., and Izuka, R. 1972. "Toxic action of anti-H.C.G. antibody to human trophoblast." *Int. J. Fertil.* **17**:65–71.

Pressman, D., and Korngold, L. 1957. "Localizing properties of anti-placental serum." *J. Immunol.* **78**:75–78.

Seegal, B. C., and Loeb, E. N. 1946. "Production of chronic glomerulonephritis in rats by injection of rabbit anti-rat-placenta serum." *J. Exp. Med.* **84**:211–222.

Stebley, R. W. 1962. "Localization in human kidney of antibodies formed in sheep against human placenta." *J. Immunol.* **88**:434–442.

Chapter 9

Nonspecific and Specific Weakening of the Maternal Immune Response During Pregnancy

As we have already seen, observations from studies on normal tropho-blast and its malignant derivative, choriocarcinoma (see Chapter 7), indi-cate that the peculiar immunologic properties of this tissue could afford a sufficient explanation for the survival to term of allogeneic fetuses in both normal and specifically sensitized mothers. There are factors operating dur-ing pregnancy, however, that could lead to both nonspecific and specific alterations of a female's capacity to become sensitized to the histocom-patibility antigens of her fetus or to express an extant sensitivity. Currently a great deal of attention is being devoted to the definition of these factors and their *modus operandi,* with considerable emphasis upon *in vitro* pro-cedures. Apart from the light this work may shed upon ancillary mecha-nisms that may protect the fetus as an allograft, it may also lead to our better understanding of immunoregulatory processes in general and their role in malignant and autoimmune diseases.

EVIDENCE FOR THE OCCURRENCE OF NONSPECIFIC WEAKENING OF THE MATERNAL IMMUNE RESPONSE DURING PREGNANCY

It has long been known that during pregnancy there is an increased production of certain hormones, notably adrenal corticosteroids, and temporary involution of lymphoid tissue, most markedly of the thymus, which in the mouse may lose 70% of its initial weight. These hormones when administered in abnormally high dosages under experimental con-ditions bring about a transient lymphocytopenia, a marked involution of lymphoid tissue, suppression of inflammation, and significant weakening of a host's reactivity to a primary allograft of skin. Progesterone and es-trogen, produced by the placenta throughout pregnancy and resulting in

119

a severalfold increase in plasma concentrations over those found in non-pregnant females, have also been shown to have immunosuppressive properties as far as skin allografts are concerned.

In women there is evidence, albeit of a less cogent nature, that suggests that pregnancy is sometimes associated with a decreased resistance to some infectious diseases such as hepatitis, smallpox, influenza, coccidiomycosis, poliomyelitis, herpes simplex, and mammary cancer. In addition there are reports of a lowered incidence of positive delayed cutaneous reactions to contact allergens and an amelioration of the symptoms of some diseases of suspected autoimmune etiology, including rheumatoid arthritis. Most of these alleged pregnancy-associated alterations pertain to T lymphocyte-mediated or -dependent reactions.

On the basis of this kind of evidence the idea that the immunological capacity of the mother undergoes a physiological change that protects the fetus from the potential dangers of sensitizing her was considered by Medawar more than 20 years ago. Support for this premise was afforded by the observation of Heslop and his colleagues at the University of Birmingham, England, that skin allografts transplanted to rabbits that were about 3 weeks' pregnant survived almost twice as long as grafts transplanted sooner or later in pregnancy or to virgin animals. This observation was interpreted as indicating that the peak period of enhanced steroid secretion occurred during the latter part of pregnancy. In women, too, there are reports that hint at some weakening of allograft reactivity during pregnancy. In mice, extensive investigations have failed to reveal any impairment of a female's reactivity to grafts of H-2 locus incompatible skin during intrastrain pregnancies, though a trivial weakening of their response to grafts confronting them with only minor alien tissue antigens is demonstrable. It is important to note that in both experimental and clinical contexts certain adrenal glucocorticoid hormones administered for prolonged periods in high dosages have the important property of being able to erase immunological memory. With one exception (see page 162), neither in the rabbit nor in any other species has it been shown that pregnancy can weaken a preexisting state of allograft immunity. At best, therefore, the increased steroid levels in the blood, to which both fetus and its placenta probably contribute, can only be regarded as affording a weak ancillary mechanism for preventing the development of maternal alloimmunity during pregnancy in a few species.

There is one additional possibility still on probation, however, raised initially by the finding that cortisone could also exercise its effect when applied topically on skin allografts at dosage levels that had little activity when administered systematically to the host rabbits. Some hormones produced by trophoblast, and normally present in relatively high concentration in association with this tissue throughout pregnancy, may suppress interaction between maternal lymphocytes, whether they be antigen-sensitive cells or actual effector cells, and the fetal trophoblast. In man two obvious candidates for this role are hormones specific for the placenta-chorionic gonadotropin (HCG) and somatomammotropin (HPL). HCG, a glycoprotein, appears in the maternal blood almost immediately after implantation and is produced in large amounts by normal trophoblast, as well as by choriocarcinoma (see Fig. 7-1). HPL, a polypeptide, is found in maternal blood after the fourth week of pregnancy and increases in concentration rapidly thereafter. Several investigators have shown that both of these hormones, when present at physiologic concentrations, significantly suppress the normal response of lymphocytes *in vitro* to phytohemagglutinin, a T cell mitogen, which is generally held to be an indication of immunocompetence.

Dr. Eugene Adcock and his colleagues at the University of Colorado Medical Center have shown, in addition, that this inhibition of the response of human lymphocytes to PHA is reversible and takes place without cytotoxicity. These investigators raised the interesting possibility that the carbohydrate moiety of HCG, which makes up 31.3% of this glycoprotein by weight, may represent surface antigen on trophoblast cells, by analogy with the fact that some glycoproteins of saliva carry ABO blood group antigens. They point out that if this is the case, a high concentration of HCG surrounding the trophoblast at implantation would block the rejection of trophoblast by maternal lymphocytes. Hormones analogous to HCG and HPL, however, have not been shown to be produced by the trophoblast of rats or of many other species. Consequently, unless equivalent hormones with similar effects on lymphocytes can be shown to be synthesized by trophoblast cells in these species, one must have serious reservations about the general validity of this interesting premise.

Dr. William J. Byrd, of the Salk Institute, has discovered that crude extracts of mouse placenta inhibit some *in vitro* parameters of immune responsiveness, including mitogen-induced transformation of immunocompetent cells, mixed leukocyte culture reactions, and the generation of cytotoxic "killer" lymphocytes when tested on lymphoid cells obtained from normal, nonpregnant animals.

Many investigators have reasoned that if a generalized depression of a pregnant female's cellular immune system contributes significantly to the nonrejection of fetal allografts, lymphocytes from pregnant women should display impaired immunologic responses *in vitro*. Although there is no doubt that pregnant women's lymphocytes do respond to PHA stimulation by DNA synthesis *in vitro*, however, there is considerable disagreement whether their level of response is similar to that of controls. The most critical and extensive investigation to date is that undertaken by Dr. Martin Carr and his associates from the University of California at San Francisco.

They have studied the dose-time response kinetics of PHA stimulation of peripheral blood lymphocytes from pregnant women. At optimum concentrations of the mitogen the responses of their lymphocytes were not impaired: Indeed, compared to controls they seemed to have *higher* levels of DNA synthesis when unstimulated and gave greater responses at suboptimal PHA concentrations and a lower peak dose response. These observations, which were most evident in the third trimester of pregnancy, suggest that a pregnant woman's lymphocytes are indeed fully competent to respond to PHA stimulation and so, by implication, are fully reactive in an immunological sense. Moreover, the findings hint that the lymphocytes at the time of harvesting were already undergoing a low level of stimulation, possibly as a consequence of the mother's exposure to alien cells or proteins of fetal origin. These conclusions are in accord with previous observations that the reactivity of lymphocytes from women at the time of delivery to cells from unrelated allogeneic donors in MLC tests is not significantly impaired. Contrary to expectations is the finding that when lymphocytes taken from women at parturition are treated with mitomycin C and used as "stimulating" cells in MLC tests, they are *less* effective than lymphocytes from normal female donors.

None of these findings excludes a role for specific or nonspecific humoral factors since maternal plasma was excluded from the *in vitro* test systems employed.

Evidence for the Occurrence of Specific Modification of the Maternal Immune Response During Pregnancy

Any specific modification of the immunological response repertoire of pregnant females must necessarily result from their exposure to antigenic material originating from their fetuses, including of course the fetal component of the placenta. The phenomenon of Rh sensitization in man provides a striking example of the facility with which active immunization can take place to antigens of one particular blood group system, the determinants of which are only expressed on erythrocytes, as a result of very small dosage fetal → maternal transplacental leakages. Placental porosity also extends to other types of cells (see Chapter 11).

Prior to reviewing the current state of knowledge concerning the actual consequences of the known or suspected presentation of fetal cellular and other antigens into the mother, let us briefly review what the theoretical possibilities are. The most obvious one is *active* sensitization of the mother with regard to the alien, paternally inherited antigens of her fetus. As far as transplantation antigens are concerned, this should readily be detectable by accelerated rejection of test grafts from the offspring or, more conveniently, from a member of the paternal strain in situations where inbred strains are available. But, as already seen, this rarely seems to take place. The second possibility, which at first sight seems less likely, is that there might be a specific *weakening* of the maternal reactivity that could be an expression of either one or other, or possibly both, of what the present authors believe to be two formally different phenomena with closely similar end points—immunological tolerance or immunological paralysis on the one hand and immunological enhancement on the other hand.

The Phenomenon of Immunological Tolerance

Immunological tolerance has been broadly defined as a state of specific *nonreactivity* to a normally effective antigenic challenge that is induced in an animal by prior exposure to the antigen concerned. The principle applies to transplantation antigens and is most readily inducible with viable suspensions of cells of the lymphohematopoietic system, although under certain conditions it can be induced by inoculation of antigenic extracts. The phenomenon of tolerance also extends to heterologous protein antigens, especially those of the blood, and to many other types of antigen. Indeed, becoming tolerant of one's *own* distinctive ingredients which are not present in lymphoid cells is probably an important developmental process which protects against the risk of autoimmunization. Tolerance is most readily induced in very young, immunologically immature animals, though by various artifices it can also be induced in adult subjects. To render an adult subject tolerant usually requires its inoculation with massive dosages of the antigen over prolonged periods, preferably in conjunction with an immunosuppressive agent, such as a cytotoxic drug, heterologous anti-lymphocyte globulin (ALG), or whole-body X irradiation. Irrespective of the age of the subject, with transplantation antigens the dose of the antigen required to induce tolerance depends on the degree of immunogenetic disparity involved—weak histocompatibility barriers being much easier to overcome than strong ones.

Apart from this "high-dosage" or "high-zone" tolerance, it is important to note that in studies conducted upon adult mice with bovine serum albumin (BSA) and with flagellin as antigen, both of which can induce tolerance at high-dosage levels, tolerance is also inducible by the administration of extremely small amounts of antigen. For example, with BSA a high-zone tolerogenic dose is of the order of 5 mg, whereas a low-zone dose of this tolerogen is 10–40 μg. There are some indications that the principle of low-zone tolerance also applies to transplantation antigens. For example, Billingham and Sparrow found that a highly significant prolongation of survival of skin allografts could be obtained in adult rabbits by prior intravenous injection of relatively small numbers (10–20 × 10⁶) of viable dissociated epidermal cells or leukocytes from the future donor. Another possible manifestation of low-dosage tolerance in transplantation immunology is the finding by Dr. Earle Owen and his associates that the daily intravenous administration of exceedingly small doses of subcellular donor liver "antigen" in saline—the equivalent of only 2500 hepatocytes—for 5 weeks prior to transplantation almost doubled the life expectancy of renal allografts from the same donor rabbit.

The essential features of tolerance are (1) It expresses itself as complete or partial highly specific unresponsiveness to an antigen. (2) It depends on a *central* inhibition of response at the level of the lymphoid tissue apparatus—there is either an induced absence or deficiency of appropriate clones of antigen-reactive cells, or their capacity to react is inhibited; (3) A state of tolerance can normally be abolished by transfer of lymphoid cells from a normal syngeneic donor to a tolerant animal, which makes good its deficiency in reactive cells. Tolerance is not transferable by means of serum; Finally, (4) lymphoid cells from an animal which has been rendered tolerant of the tissue antigens of a donor of an unrelated, major locus histoincompatible strain do not react in MLC tests with cells from that strain.

THE PHENOMENON OF IMMUNOLOGICAL ENHANCEMENT

Immunological enhancement may be defined as a highly specific frustration of both the antigenic stimulus and the hosts' cellular immune response, mediated by humoral isoantibody. When adult animals are confronted by allografts, they normally respond in two distinct ways to the alien histocompatibility gene products on the cell surfaces: (1) By the generation of a population of "effector" or "killer" T lymphocytes which circulate in the bloodstream and, in some as yet incompletely understood manner, are capable of infiltrating and destroying the allografts which incited their formation by a so-called cellular immunity. These effector cells can also destroy target cells *in vitro* in the absence of humoral antibodies. (2) By the synthesis of humoral antibodies of a variety of types, which are also capable of reacting with antigenic determinants on the surfaces of the target cells, both *in vivo* and *in vitro* In the presence of complement, some of these antibodies have a cytopathogenic action. This action varies in severity depending on the histological type of the target cell, lymphoid and myeloid cells being especially susceptible and sarcoma cells being highly resistant. Variation in the density of antigenic determinants on the target cell membranes is probably responsible for this differential susceptibility.

In the case of certain kinds of tumor allograft, as well as some normal tissues and renal and heart allografts in some species, it has been shown that the presence of a high titer of serum antibodies may dramatically weaken the host's capacity to react against and destroy them. This immunosuppressive effect, which is highly specific, "enhances" or prolongs the survival of the graft. The requisite levels of antibody may be obtained in two ways: (1) by active immunization of the host by repeated inoculation with homogenates, desiccates, or other rather crude, nonliving preparations, and in some circumstances even with living grafts from the donor strain of the future allograft (active enhancement), or (2) by passive transfer of these antibodies to a normal host. Passive enhancement can also take place naturally from an actively immunized (i.e., enhanced) mother to her perinatal offspring across the placenta or via the milk.

As in the case of tolerance, there are marked differences in the ease with which enhancement is procurable and its completeness, depending on the genetic relationship between donor and host and the kind of tissue or organ allograft involved. Where strong transplantation antigens are involved, the cellular immune response incited by many types of grafts, including skin, can usually override any prior enhancing treatment. In many instances apparently minor variations in the enhancing protocol may prove important in determining whether an animal's capacity to reject an allograft is weakened or unaffected. The fact that animals that can reject allografts may, with further treatment, become unresponsive suggests that the difference between an enhanced and an immune state may be a very subtle one.

Interest in immunological enhancement has been greatly heightened by the finding that intravenous injection of rats and rabbits with a relatively small dosage of donor spleen cells, followed by transfer of specific antiserum or even by transfer of antiserum alone, will prolong the survival of major locus incompatible renal transplants, but not skin grafts, for very long periods. Once the enhanced allograft has become established, it appears to furnish a continuous source of appropriate antigens to stimulate and maintain production of enhancing antibody by the host—i.e., "auto-enhancement."

Since so much of our early knowledge of transplantation immunology has been based upon the study of orthotopic allografts of skin, the skin allograft is usually made the standard of comparison for the successful feto-placental allograft. Since renal allografts in rats and rabbits (and liver allografts in rats and pigs) are far less exacting in their immunogenetic requirements for success than skin allografts, however, they are obviously more appropriate allografts with which to compare fetuses. Whereas skin allografts appear to incite a cellular immunity more readily than a humoral immunity and are relatively resistant to enhancing procedures, the opposite pertains to the renal and other organ allografts mentioned, as well as to the fetuses.

Cellular immunity is suppressed in rats bearing long-surviving renal allografts since these organs are not infiltrated with lymphocytes and the animals will accept skin allografts from the donor strain. This suppression of cellular immunity is reversible, however, since spleen cells taken from animals bearing long-surviving renal allografts are capable of mounting graft-versus-host reactions if injected into appropriate F_1 hybrid hosts. Furthermore, lymphoid cells from these animals are capable of responding to donor-type stimulator lymphocytes in MLC tests.

Although there is no doubt that enhancement is an antibody-mediated phenomenon, final agreement as to how the IgG class antibodies responsible mediate this unresponsiveness has yet to be achieved. Two contributory processes appear to be (1) combination of the pertinent antibodies with the antigenic determinant sites on the cell comprising the allograft, thus "masking" them from the attentions of specific antigen-sensitive lymphocytes and so interfering with both the elicitation (following a "recognition" process) and the fulfillment of the host's cellular immune response—i.e., both "afferent" and "efferent" inhibition; and (2) by some kind of central inhibitory action on the host's immunological response machinery by antibodies, or more likely by antigen-antibody complexes, impairing the development of cellular immunity, and possibly also by interfering with its expression.

Recent studies on the enhancement of renal allografts in rats by Drs. Hildemann and Mullen, in conjunction with the findings of other workers, have indicated that the effectiveness of enhancing antibodies in prolonging the survival of allografts increases as the immunogenetical disparity between donor and host decreases—i.e., it is much easier to overcome minor histoincompatibilities than major ones by means of enhancing procedures, as previously shown to be the case with the induction of immunological tolerance.

Drs. Karl and Ingegerd Hellström, and various associates, have employed an *in vitro* test for sensitized lymphocytes (which turns upon their capacity to prevent allogeneic target cells from forming colonies and so by implication killing them) to study (1) mice and dogs rendered tolerant and chimeric in adult life by whole-body irradiation followed by transfusion of alien bone marrow cells, (2) mice rendered tolerant by neonatal inoculation with alien cells, and (3) intrinsically tolerant tetraparental mice. They claim on the basis of their test that in all of these various types of "tolerant" subjects, "immune" lymphocytes are present that are capable of destroying genetically appropriate target cells *in vitro.* However serum factors believed to be antibodies are also present *in vivo* that can block this lymphocyte activity *in vitro,* and these workers suggest that it may be similarly active *in vivo*. These observations are in accord with previous findings of Dr. Guy Voisin and his colleagues in Paris that the serum of mice rendered tolerant by neonatal inoculation of allogeneic cells often contains hemagglutinins specific for donor strain cells and manifests "enhancing" activity on transfer to appropriate hosts. On the basis of these and other observations the Hellströms have suggested that some examples of tolerance of allogeneic cells and tissues may in fact be due to the presence of serum factors that can block lymphocyte reactivity rather than to a specific central failure of the immune response machinery. As far as transplantation antigens are concerned, a variety of observations make it difficult to accept the premise that enhancement is responsible for the much studied neonatally induced tolerance of skin allografts in mice and rats. For example, in most investigators' experience, lymphocytes removed from such tolerant animals retain their unresponsiveness when subjected to both *in vitro* and *in vivo* tests. By contrast, as already mentioned, lymphoid cells from passively enhanced rats bearing renal allografts of long-standing display normal immunologic reactivity, both *in vivo* and *in vitro,* against cells having the same alien genetic origin as the renal allografts.

As Hildemann and Mullen have recently suggested, however, tolerance and enhancement are both highly specific immunosuppressive processes that could coexist in one and the same unresponsive individual. To discuss the interrelationships of these two important phenomena further at this juncture would serve no useful purpose.

The Phenomenon of Graft-induced Specific Unresponsiveness

A state of complete or partial specific unresponsiveness of allogeneic grafts of skin can sometimes be induced in adult mice and rats simply by prior, long-term exposure to allografts of ovary, testis, and neonatal skin transplanted orthotopically. In the Syrian hamster, grafts of cheek pouch skin are also effective in this respect. In general, grafts of these various types are immunogenically inferior to grafts of adult skin from similar donors. Usually this phenomenon of graft-induced "tolerance" only expresses itself in situations in which relatively minor degrees of histoincompatibility are involved. Since this method of obtaining unresponsiveness in adult hosts clearly cannot entail systemic exposure of the host to large amounts of antigen, it seemed reasonable, at least provisionally, to regard low-zone tolerance as the underlying mechanism. As a result of our recent better understanding of the phenomenon of immunological enhancement, however, it is obvious that this could also account for at least some of the instances of graft-induced tolerance.

Drs. Stephen Wachtel and Willys K. Silvers of the University of Pennsylvania have carefully analyzed the state of tolerance that skin allografts from neonatal C3H strain mice can confer upon adult CBA strain hosts, and this may extend to subsequent grafts of adult skin from the same donor strain. Their findings implicate "passenger" leukocytes carried over in the blood vessels of the neonatal grafts as the principal tolerogens: Removal of these cells prior to transplantation, for example by X irradiation, deprives the grafts of their longevity. Furthermore it was found that the continued presence of the neonatal C3H skin grafts was not necessary to maintain tolerance in the CBA hosts—this finding was consistent with evidence that CBA males bearing long-term grafts of C3H skin from neonatal donors were chimeric with respect to their leukocytes. A further indication that passenger leukocytes that escaped from the skin grafts into the host's vasculature were the prime movers in tolerance induction was the finding that subcutaneous inoculation of leukocytes from neonatal C3H donors into CBA male hosts occasionally resulted in unresponsiveness to subsequent grafts of adult C3H skin. Administration of leukocytes from *adult* C3H donors, however, nearly always sensitized their hosts.

Another familiar and fairly well-studied example of graft-induced unresponsiveness relates to the Y-linked, male-specific transplantation antigen as it is expressed in the C57BL/6 strain of mice. Because of the association of this antigen with cells from syngeneic males, females reject grafts from these donors within about 25 days; however, the majority of females will accept skin grafts from neonatal C57 male donors. About 50% of the females that have tolerated grafts of neonatal male skin for 50 days are found to have become unresponsive to grafts from *adult* male donors. Recent analysis of this particular example of graft-induced unresponsiveness indicates that passenger cells are not responsible for it. The unresponsive females are not demonstrably chimeric and persistence of the unresponsive state *is* dependent on the continued presence of the graft of neonatal male skin. In the light of this and other evidence a cogent argument can now be made out for enhancement as the phenomenon involved.

The well-documented observation discussed in detail in Chapter 11 that, in humans, leukocyte antibodies are frequently present in maternal serum following a first and usually after two or more pregnancies affords indirect evidence of the occurrence or frequency of fetal → maternal transmission of leukocytes during gestation since the antigens concerned are not present on erythrocytes. Whether these antigens are associated with trophoblast cells in an effective form remains an open question (see page 102). Since multiparous women can only form antibodies against alien, paternally inherited leukocytes of their fetuses, these antibodies are necessarily of limited specificity, sometimes being capable of recognizing only a single antigen. Such individuals have proved to be an invaluable source of sera for tissue typing since most of the serologically detectable antigenic determinants referred to as "leukocyte antigens" are in fact histocompatibility antigens. It is interesting to note that these antibodies persist at relatively high titers in the sera of multiparous women for many years after their final pregnancy.

In mice, too, antibodies detectable as hemagglutinins and also corresponding to histocompatibility determinants that the fetuses inherited from their fathers appear in the serum of multiparous females. The observation that repeated matings of sterile females with unrelated males fail to incite the formation of these antibodies indicates that the fetuses are the source of this antigenic stimulus. There remains, of course, the remote possibility that the occasional baby that mothers eat might have been the source. In rats, by contrast, multiparity by Ag-B locus incompatible males does not lead to the appearance of hemagglutinating antibodies in the females, though there is evidence that it does evoke the formation of isoantibodies with enhancing properties.

The evidence so far presented in this section suggests that, at least in some species, during pregnancy fetal cells do normally cross the placenta and enter the maternal circulation as well as the lymphatics draining the gravid uterus since the regional nodes undergo hypertrophy during pregnancies by allogeneic males. Indeed this lymph node adenopathy, which is evident long before parturition, indicates that the latter event is not the time of significant exposure of mothers to cells of their progeny. The parity-induced specific weakening of allograft reactivity that results from this exposure will be discussed (see page 160).

Concept of Immunological Inertia of Viviparity

In a series of publications, Dr. J. Maxwell Anderson of the University of Glasgow has presented the results of infant to maternal skin grafting experiments on outbred stocks of four different species: armadillos, dogs, sheep, and principally rats. On the basis of the findings he postulated that a state of specific immunological hypoactivity or "immunological inertia" between mother and fetus occurs during pregnancy, having "special features which distinguish it from tolerance, paralysis or desensitization." He observed that skin grafts from very young offspring lived significantly longer on their mothers than grafts from older offspring and interpreted this as indicative that the mother's inertia toward her offspring's tissue antigens is a temporary and gradually waning phenomenon. The prompt rejection of skin allografts from newborn rats transplanted to unrelated postpartum rats was construed as evidence of the specificity of this phenomenon.

The findings of other investigators that the immunogenicity of infant rodent's skin is demonstrably inferior to that of skin from older donors, especially where nonmajor histocompatibility locus differences are concerned, however, suggests an alternative and much more likely explanation of the alleged inertia of the mother. Furthermore, Anderson's evidence that his phenomenon is specific is totally unconvincing since, in outbred populations, one would expect that grafts from their own offspring would survive longer on mothers than would grafts from unrelated donors of similar age.

Experiments are currently in progress in the authors' laboratory to evaluate the effect of immunogenetically alien pregnancies on the immunologic reactivity of female rats, using inbred strains. Female Fischer rats have been grafted 10 days postpartum with skin from (Fischer × DA)F₁ hybrid donors, after one, two to four, and five to eight pregnancies by DA strain males (see Fig. 9-1). It was found that, irrespective of the age of the donors, (1) Virgin females (controls) consistently rejected their hy-

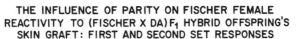

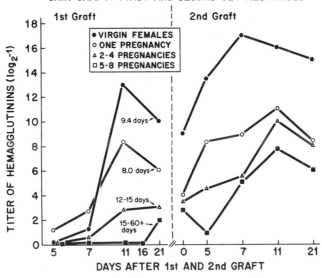

Fig. 9-1. Influence of numbers of pregnancies in female Fischer strain rats mated to DA strain males on (a) The median survival times of (FI × DA)F₁ hybrid skin allografts transplanted to them 10 days after birth of the final litter in the series and (b) the titers of hemagglutinins incited by these allografts. The hemagglutining titers following transplantation of second-set skin allografts are also recorded. These findings show that whereas uniparous females rejected their test grafts significantly more rapidly than virgin females (indicative of weak transplantation immunity), multiparous females displayed hyporeactivity to their grafts that increased with parity. It will be noted that parity progressively impaired their capacity to produce hemagglutinins in response to the skin allografts.

brid test grafts within 9 days of grafting and developed high titers of hemagglutinins (both 19-S and 7-S antibodies) during rejection of first-set grafts and even higher titers during rejection of second-set skin grafts. (2) By contrast, the intensity of the reactivity of primiparous females to their test grafts was somewhat greater than that of the controls, as evidenced by the shortened survival times; however, their ability to produce hemagglutinating antibodies during rejection of both first- and second-set skin allografts was significantly depressed. (3) Multiparous females, on the other hand, rejected their grafts much more slowly, some grafts surviving for upward of 60 days, and the animals developed a very feeble antibody response to both first- and second-set skin allografts. (4) This apparent immunologic hypoactive state did not extend to grafts from a third, unrelated donor strain, such as BN or Lewis.

That the fetal antigen responsible for inducing this maternal hyporeactivity derived from the trophoblast was evidenced by the observation that single as well as sequential allogeneic grafts of pure trophoblast, derived from ectoplacental cones, inserted beneath the renal capsules of virgin females also resulted in a specifically impaired reactivity to skin allografts. The observation that females whose para-aortic nodes were excised prior to allogeneic pregnancies failed to become hyporeactive suggests that during allogeneic pregnancies a specific factor, possibly a "blocking antibody," is produced in these lymphoid organs.

These findings indicate that a specific factor(s), possibly a blocking antibody not measured by hemagglutination, appears during pregnancy and is capable of facilitating in the mother the induction of a specific state of immunological unresponsiveness toward solid tissue allografts having the same genetic makeup as the fetuses. However, this "frustrating" influence of what is probably a blocking antibody on maternal cellular immune reactivity does not entail a permanent, irreversible suppression of specific maternal, antigen-reactive lymphocytes. This conclusion is based upon the finding that when lymphoid cells were harvested from multiparous females and transferred to normal syngeneic or F_1 hybrid hosts, they were rapidly released from their *in vivo* restraints and behaved just like populations of cells from sensitized donors, adoptively immunizing and inciting graft-versus-host reactions, respectively.

EVIDENCE THAT PREGNANCY CAN CAUSE
A CELLULAR IMMUNITY DIRECTED
AGAINST FETAL TISSUE ANTIGENS

As previously mentioned, nearly all grafting tests performed on female mice and, to a limited extent, upon females of other species parous by allogeneic males, if they revealed any alteration in response at all, gave evidence of a *weakening* of reactivity toward these antigens the females had been exposed to during pregnancy. This led to the very reasonable conclusion that their ability to undertake cellular immune responses had been partially abrogated, probably by the action of blocking or enhancing antibodies.

That the failure of allogeneic fetuses to incite cellular immune responses on the part of their mothers was more apparent than real was first suggested by the work of Sörén. He harvested lymphoid cells from female mice that had been outcrossed to males of an H-2 locus incompatible strain (CBA or C57 females mated with A strain males) and injected them into the neonatal F_1 hybrid progeny of these matings. More intense graft-versus-host reactions (as evidenced by greater spleen indices) were incited by these inocula than by similar injections of lymphoid cells from virgin female donors of the same strain.

Recognizing the importance of removing the lymphocytes from the milieu of pregnant or parous females (to isolate them as far as possible from enhancing antibodies or other immunosuppressant agents) before testing their reactivity against the alien antigens of their fetuses, other investigators have now confirmed and extended Sörén's work.

In experiments conducted upon mice and rats it has been shown that

1. Lymphoid cells taken from females parous by major-locus incompatible males and transferred to syngeneic normal males and females are capable of adoptively immunizing the latter with regard to subsequent test skin allografts from the paternal strain.

2. Lymphoid cells from females parous by allogeneic but major-locus compatible males, injected into the feet of young F_1 hybrid hosts, incite significantly greater degrees of hypertrophy of the draining popliteal lymph nodes (a measure of GVH reactivity) than cells from virgin donors of the same strain.

3. In the rat, Beer and his associates have found that, following a single pregnancy by a Lewis male, Fischer females do reject allografts of Lewis skin significantly faster than virgin Fischer females.

It is important to note that when graft-versus-host reactivity was employed to test the immunological status of maternal lymphocytes, positive results were only forthcoming if the mothers had undergone several hetero-specific pregnancies, probably because of the relative insensitivity of the test system and the fact that sensitization was progressive.

In man, too, it has now been shown the multiparity leads to maternal hypersensitivity to fetal, presumably paternally inherited, antigens. Rocklin and co-workers from Harvard Medical College used an *in vitro* correlate of cellular hypersensitivity, i.e., the *macrophage migration inhibition assay,* to study the immunological status of the mother's lymphocytes *vis-à-vis* those of her infant. This assay measures the elaboration of a soluble material, known as *migration inhibition factor* or *MIF* (which belongs to the class of lymphocytic mediators of delayed hypersensitivity known as *lymphokines*), from sensitized lymphocytes after stimulation with the specific antigen. In the present study, mothers' peripheral blood lymphocytes were exposed to those of their offspring at a ratio of 5:1 *in vitro* in a medium that contained neither serum nor antibiotics. The cell-free supernatants were then harvested over a 3-day period, concentrated, and assayed for their capacity to inhibit the migration of macrophages from normal guinea pigs from the open ends of glass capillary tubes. The results were very striking: Although lymphocytes from women who had undergone one or two pregnancies failed to produce MIF, those from subjects of three or more pregnancies consistently produced this factor when exposed to their infants' cells but not when exposed to cells from unrelated donors. No evidence of MIF production was obtained when infants' cells were mixed at a 5:1 ratio with maternal lymphocytes, suggesting that the infants had not been sensitized against maternal antigens. This result is scarcely surprising in view of the several pregnancies required to sensitize their mothers.

No attempt was made to determine the influence of pretreating infants' lymphocytes with maternal serum before using them to stimulate MIF production by maternal lymphocytes. This might have yielded evidence of the presence of inhibitory agents.

REFERENCES

Adcock, E. W., Teasdale, F., August, C. S., Cox, C., Meschia, G., Battaglia, F. C., and Naughton, M. A. 1973. "Human chorionic gonadotropin: Its possible role in maternal lymphocyte suppression." *Science* **181**: 845–847.

Anderson, J. M. 1971. "Transplantation—Nature's successes." *Lancet* **ii**:1077–1082.

Andresen, R. H., and Monroe, C. W. 1962. "Experimental study of the behavior of adult human skin homografts during pregnancy." *Am. J. Obstet. Gynecol.* **84**:1096–1100.

Beer, A. E., and Billingham, R. E. 1971. "Immunobiology of mammalian reproduction." *Adv. Immunol.* **14**:1–84.

Beer, A. E., and Billingham, R. E. 1974. "Host responses to intra-uterine tissue, cellular and fetal allografts." *J. Reprod. Fertil. Suppl.* **21**:59–83.

Billingham, R. E. 1974. "The phenomenon of immunological tolerance and its possible role in development." In *Concepts of development* (J. Lash and J. R. Whittaker, ed.). Sinauer Associates, Stamford, Conn., pp. 272–292.

Billingham, R. E., Krohn, P. L., and Medawar, P. B. 1951. "Effect of locally applied cortisone acetate on survival of skin homografts in rabbits." *Brit. Med. J.* ii:1049–1053.

Billingham, R. E., and Sparrow, E. M. 1955. "The effect of prior intravenous injections of dissociated epidermal cells and blood on the survival of skin homografts in rabbits." *J. Embryol. Exp. Morphol.* 3:266–285.

Breyere, E. J., and Burhoe, S. O., 1963. "Nature of partial tolerance induced by parity." *J. Natl. Cancer Inst.* 31:179–188.

Breyere, E. J., and Spiess, P. J. 1973. "Reduction of preexisting transplantation immunity by specific pregnancy." *Transplantation* 15:413–415.

Carr, M. C., Stites, D. P., and Fudenberg, H. H., 1973. "Cellular immune aspects of the human fetal maternal relationship. II. *In vitro* response of gravida lymphocytes to phytohemagglutinin." *Cell. Immunol.* 8: 448–454.

Cepellini, R., Bonnard, G. D., Coppo, F., Miggiano, V. C., Pospisil, M., Curtoni, E. S., and Pellegrino, M. 1971. "Mixed leukocyte cultures and HL-A antigens. I. Reactivity of young fetuses, newborns, and mothers at delivery." *Tranpl. Proc.* 3:58–70.

Currie, G. A. 1970. "The conceptus as an allograft: Immunological reactivity of the mother." *Proc. Roy. Soc. Med.* 63:61–64.

French, M. E., and Batchelor, J. R. 1972. "Enhancement of renal allografts in rats and man." *Transpl. Rev.* 13:115–141.

Goodlin, R. C., and Herzenberg, L. A. 1964. "Pregnancy induced hemagglutinins to parental H-2 antigens in multiparous mice." *Transplantation* 2:357–361.

Hellström, K. E., and Hellström, I. 1972. "The role of serum factors ("blocking antibodies") as mediators of immunological non-reactivity to cellular antigens. In *Ontogeny of acquired immunity*. Ciba Foundation Symposium. Elsevier, Excerpta Medica, North-Holland, pp. 133–143.

Heslop, R. W., Krohn, P. L., and Sparrow, E. M. 1954. "Effect of pregnancy on survival of skin homografts in rabbits." *J. Endocrinol.* 14:325–332.

Hildemann, W. H., and Mullen, Y. 1973. "The weaker the histoincompatibility, the greater the effectiveness of specific immunoblocking antibodies: A new immunogenetic rule of transplantation." *Transpl. Proc.* 5:617–620.

Jeekel, J. 1973. "The behavior of male skin grafts in isogenic postpartum female mice." *Transplantation* 16:570–578.

Jenkins, D. M., Acres, M. G., Peters, J., and Riley, J. 1972. "Human chorionic gonadotropin and the fetal allograft." *Am. J. Obstet. Gynecol.* **114**: 13–15.

Kaliss, N., and Dagg, M. 1964. "Immune response engendered in mice by multiparity." *Transplantation* **2**:416–425.

Kaliss, N., and Rubinstein, P. 1968. "Absence of correlation between presence of pregnancy-induced hemagglutinins and stage of pregnancy in mice." *Proc. Soc. Exp. Biol. Med.* **128**:1214–1217.

Kaye, M. D., and Jones, W. R. 1971. "Effect of human chorionic gonadotropin on *in vitro* lymphocyte transformation." *Am. J. Obstet. Gynecol.* **109**: 1029–1031.

Maroni, E. S., and DeSousa, M. A. B. 1973. "The lymphoid organs during pregnancy in the mouse. A comparison between a syngeneic and an allogeneic mating." *Clin. Exp. Immunol.* **13**:107–124.

Maroni, E. S., and Parrott, D. M. 1973. "Progressive increase in cell mediated immunity against paternal transplantation antigens in parous mice after multiple pregnancies." *Clin. Exp. Immunol.* **13**:253–262.

Medawar, P. B. 1953. "Some immunological and endocrinological problems raised by the evolution of viviparity in vertebrates." *In* Symp. Soc. Exp. Biol., No. 11, *Evolution.* Academic Press, New York, pp. 320–338.

Medawar, P. B. 1969. "Immunosuppressive agents, with special reference to antilymphocyte serum." *Proc. Roy. Soc.* (London) Series B, **174**:155–172.

Munroe, J. S. 1971. "Progesteroids as immunosuppressive agents." *J. Reticuloendothel. Soc.* **9**:361–375.

Nelson, J. H., and Hall, J. E. 1964. "Studies on the thymolymphatic system in humans." *Am. J. Obstet. Gynecol.* **90**:482–484.

Payne, R. 1962. "The development and persistence of leukoagglutinins in parous women." *Blood* **19**:411–424.

Porter, J. B., and Breyere, E. J. 1964. "Studies on source of antigenic stimulation in induction of tolerance by parity." *Transplantation* **2**:246–250.

Rocklin, R. E., Zuckerman, J. E., Alpert, E., and David, J. R. 1973. "Effect of multiparity on human maternal hypersensitivity to foetal antigen." *Nature* **241**:130–131.

Simmons, R. L., Ozerkis, A. J., Butsch, D. W., and Russell, P. S. 1967. "The immunologic problem of pregnancy. III. Effect of pregnancy on survival of adult and neonatal skin grafts." *Am. J. Obstet. Gynecol* **99**: 266–270.

Snell, G. D. 1970. "Immunologic enhancement." *Surg., Gynecol., Obstet.* **130**: 1109–1119.

Sören, L. 1967. "Immunological reactivity of lymphocytes in multiparous females after strain specific matings." *Nature* **213**:621–622.

Van Rood, J. J., van Leeuwen, A., and Eernisse, J. G. 1959. "Leucocyte antibodies in sera of pregnant women." *Vox Sang.* (Basel) **4**:427–444.

Wachtel, S. S., and Silvers, W. K. 1972. "The role of passenger leukocytes in the anomalous survival of neonatal skin grafts in mice." *J. Exp. Med.* **135**:388–404.

Weigle, W. O. 1971. "Immunologic unresponsiveness." In *Immunobiology* (R. A. Good and D. W. Fisher, ed.). Sinauer Associates, Stamford, Conn., pp. 123–134.

Chapter 10

Immunologic Consequences of Natural
Fetal-Fetal Vascular Anastomoses
and Exchange of Cells

For more than 2000 years cattle breeders have been aware that a female calf, twin-born with a male, is nearly always deficient in its sexual development and incapable of reproduction, though to outward appearance it may be perfectly normal—the so-called freemartin. Since these females represent genetic females whose reproductive system has developed in a male direction, they have attracted the attention of embryologists and endocrinologists interested in the problem of sex differentiation. In 1916 F. R. Lillie in America and Keller and Tandler in Germany independently discovered, at least in part, the cause of the freemartin condition when they found that in order for the freemartin condition to occur there had to be an anastomosis of blood vessels between the chorions of the hetero-sexual twins. For reasons that have yet to be elucidated, in all multiple pregnancies in cattle, placental fusion nearly always occurs very early in embryonic life, allowing the establishment of interembryonic vascular anastomoses through which blood is exchanged. From this it was con-cluded that, when male fetuses are gestated co-twin with females, fetal testicular hormones of the males, gaining access to the circulation of the females, divert the normal development of their sexual organs in a male direction. A lot of unsuccessful attempts ensued, by Lillie and others, to reproduce with appropriate hormones in a variety of laboratory animals what takes place in freemartins naturally.

Another immunologically more interesting attribute that the freemartin shares with similar sexed dizygotic cattle twins emerged in the early 1940's. A group of immunogeneticists working at the University of Wisconsin showed that twin cattle have identical blood types much more frequently than expected on the basis of the frequency of identical twins. Subse-quently, on the basis of differential immune hemolysis tests, Dr. Ray D. Owen showed that most twin cattle are born with, and may retain through-out life, a stable though variable mixture of their own erythrocytes with

137

erythrocytes belonging to the cellular heritage of their co-twins. Evidently the twins exchange blood in fetal life through the anastomoses of their placental blood vessels. Since the chimeric state lasts far beyond the life-span of an erythrocyte, and may be permanent, it followed that red cell *precursors,* as well as red cells, must have been exchanged in the fetal cross-transfusion and have successfully established themselves in the tissues of the opposite twin.

Influenced by Owen's observation, Burnet and Fenner in 1950 pro-pounded a theory of antibody formation that included the prediction of the phenomenon of immunological tolerance—i.e., that if embryos are exposed to antigenic substances, their ability to react against these same substances when they grow up would be abolished or at least impaired. In the early 1950's Medawar and his associates showed that most dizygotic cattle twins would accept skin grafts from each other but not from their parents or from siblings of separate birth or from unrelated third parties. Once the connection between Owen's discovery of chimerism and this ob-servation of highly specific allograft acceptance or tolerance was appreci-ated, experiments were successfully launched to reproduce in the labora-tory, initially in mice and chickens, the state of affairs that occurs as a natural accident in twin cattle.

Natural erythrocyte chimerism is not restricted to multiple births in cattle. In 1953, when a Mrs. McK in England donated blood, it was found to comprise a mixture of A (39%) and O (61%) cells. When asked if she were a twin, this lady replied, somewhat surprised, that her twin brother had died 25 years previously at the age of 3 months. That the O cells were genetically her own was established by the fact that she secreted O (H) antigens in her saliva but not A antigen. Mrs. McK was feminine in appearance and has several children. To date a total of nine sets of chimera twins have been reported, indicating the rarity of this condition in man. Apart from being chimeras with respect to their erythro-cytes, chimerism at the level of their polymorphs, lymphocytes, and platelet precursors has also been established. The fertility of both the males and females of the male-female pairs is beyond question, and in one instance tolerance of histocompatibility antigens has been established on the basis of the acceptance of mutually exchanged skin grafts.

In all the human chimeras studied so far it has been found that the natural isohemagglutinins corresponding to their "alien" red cell moiety are absent. For example, Mrs. McK is of blood type O and her serum con-tains anti-B but no anti-A. This deficiency presumably reflects the fact that her early and subsequent continuous exposure to her brother's A-type red cells and their precursor stem cells rendered and maintained her tol-erance of this antigen.

Marmosets nearly always give birth to fraternal twins between which, as Wislocki demonstrated in 1939, vascular anastomoses are established very early in embryonic life as a consequence of chorionic fusion. This has also been shown to result in chimerism with regard to erythrocytes, leukocytes, and indeed all components of the lymphohematopoietic tissue system as well as skin graft tolerance. As in man, however, female marmosets that develop co-twin with males are perfectly normal and fertile. The biological significance of this harmless natural, consistent, synchorial vascular anastomosis in marmosets awaits explanation. In an immunologic sense the resultant state of mutual tolerance of each others' tissue antigens in these dissimilar twins might be regarded as disadvantageous since it reduces the total spectrum of antigenic specificities against which each can react. The fact that cross-reactivity exists between transplantation antigens and antigenic determinants of certain microorganisms adds some cogency to this line of reasoning.

Although very rare, chimerism in bisexual twins has also been reported and investigated in several sets of sheep twins and one set of goat twins, in both of which species the females were freemartins.

In all of these species, apart from demonstration of erythrocyte chimerism, the peripheral blood leukocytes have been shown to be chimeric by means of sex chromatin (i.e., Barr bodies) and/or sex chromosome analyses. In both cattle and human chimeras, evidence has been forthcoming that the relative proportions of the two antigenically different types of erythrocyte may change with time, and in cattle at least, "hybrid"-type erythrocytes may appear. For example, Dr. W. M. Stone and co-workers at the University of Wisconsin reported a case in cattle where the blood of one chimeric twin, when it was 3 years old, contained two red cell types, 10% corresponding to his own genotype and 90% to the genotype of his co-twin. At 8 years of age, three blood types were identifiable. of erythrocyte may change with time, and in cattle at least, "hybrid"-type represented 96% of the population. The authors believe that the "hybrid" cell type, which seemed to have a distinct selective advantage, must have resulted from "matings" between the two genetically distinct types of hematopoietic stem cells present. Similar situations have been subsequently reported by Drs. J. H. Turner and Donald Hutchinson of the University of Pittsburgh in human infants born after an intrauterine fetal blood transfusion for Rh isoimmunization.

In cattle the proportion of one population of erythrocytes in one twin is usually the same as in its co-twin, so that the predominant red cell population does not necessarily correspond to the animal's own genotype. In the marmoset Dr. N. Gengozian and his co-workers have shown that in bisexual twins the proportion of male cells in one twin is the same as in the co-twin and that there is an apparent selectivity for male cells in *all* marmosets, irrespective of their sex; the mean ratio of male to female cells is 1.36. In human chimeric twin pairs the proportion of the two types of erythrocytes in the two individuals may be similar or different.

Confirmation that freemartins in cattle are indeed genetically female was forthcoming from sex chromatin studies as well as from chromosome analyses. Apart from hematological elements it seems that other cell types are also exchanged between cattle twins. Ohno and his associates have studied newborn bisexual twins in cattle and although they could find no evidence of chimerism in the atrophic ovaries of the freemartins, they did find typical female cells in the testes of their co-twins. Other investigators have noted the presence of ovotestes in some freemartins that may have resulted from the exchange of primordial germs cells. In marmosets, Benirschke and Brownhill also obtained suggestive evidence of germ cell chimerism in the testes of males born co-twin with females. Indeed, it seems likely that the abnormalities of the freemartin may be due to the transfer of *cellular* components from the male gonads rather than hormones.

The striking discrepancy between the consistent normality of development and the fertility of female chimeras co-twin with males in man and marmosets and the high incidence of abnormalities in female chimeras co-twin with males in cattle has yet to be resolved. One explanation put forward is that androgens may be handled differently in these species. Human and marmoset placentas possess enzymes that can convert androgens to estrogens, whereas the bovine placenta is unable to do this. Most of the placental estrogen in man is derived from androgen precursors in the fetus. It may therefore be that the androgen levels in fetal calf blood are higher than those in the blood of fetal primates and effect the masculinization.

Another suggestion, put forward by Witschi, is that the testis in male cattle twins produces a factor that suppresses the development of the cortex of the female gonad, allowing the medulla to develop into a testis. This, he postulated, then produces a second factor, known as an arrhenogen, which suppresses the development of the Mullerian duct system in the female and masculinizes the external genitalia.

MONOZYGOTISM HÉTÉROCARYOTE

In 1961, Dr. Jerome Lejeune and his associates in France discovered the first example of a new type of twinning, which they described as "monozygotism hétérocaryote." These twins are monozygotic on the basis of their blood groups and mutual acceptance of each others' grafts, etc., but they do not have identical karyotypes. As Race and Sanger colorfully put it, "the accident is due to aneuploidy at some postzygotic cell division preceding the laying down of the keels of the twins in their primitive streaks."

The first pair of twins of this type described comprised an XO female suffering from Turner's syndrome and a normal XY male. Here the aneu-poloidy had occurred in the subsequent cell division of an XY zygote. Loss of the Y chromosome was responsible for the XO female.

Pairs of monozygotic twins have been found in which both members of each pair were mosaic XO/XX but one member of the pair was normal and the other displayed serious abnormality. The chromosomal mosaicism often observed in the peripheral blood leukocytes of both normal and ab-normal heterokaryote twin pairs is due to intrauterine exchange of hema-topoietic stem cells.

THE PHENOMENON OF DISPERMY

In 1962 in Seattle a young girl was discovered whose left eye was hazel and right eye was brown. Although her cultured leukocytes were euploid, about half were XX and half were XY. She was also chimeric with respect to her red cells. At laparotomy she was found to have a normal ovary on one side and an ovotestis, containing both ovarian follicles and seminiferous tubules, on the other side. Skin from the left side of her abdo-men contained mainly XX cells, whereas that from the right side contained predominantly XY cells. The only possible explanation of this situation is that *two* different sperm succeeded in contributing their quotas of genetic information to the zygote either (1) as a result of an original ovum, penetrated by the two spermatozoa, dividing to produce two identical nuclei, each of which was fertilized, or (2) by one sperm fertilizing the egg nucleus and the other fertilizing the second polar body that is near the egg cell at this time. Since the chromosome complement of the nucleus of the second polar body is not necessarily identical with that of the egg nucleus, this allows the possibility of a double genetic contribution from the mother as well as from the father. Once the two sperms have fertilized two nuclei, the two resultant zygotes stay together to produce a single chimera.

At least eight members of this rare class of dispermic, mosaic indi-viduals have so far been reported. They can be regarded as a fusion of twins dissimilar with regard to their father's genetic contribution but either identical or dissimilar with regard to their mother's contribution. Since the two sperm do not have to come from the same male, it is possible, as Race and Sanger facetiously point out, that a few very rare individuals may have been born of one mother yet sired by *two* fathers.

TETRAPARENTAL MICE

Chimeric mice and rats can be produced by the fusion *in vitro* of the blastomeres from two genetically different blastulae and subsequent transfer to the uterus of a pseudopregnant surrogate mother. Such embryos of binary origin will develop to maturity as single "tetra-parental" individuals. The fused zygotes may differ from one another at major and other histocompatibility loci. They are chimeric and may exhibit mosaicism in many different tissues including blood, spleen, and skin, and they are usually fully tolerant of skin grafts—so-called *intrinsic* immunological tolerance—from donors of the strains that provided the blastocysts, though they can reject grafts from unrelated donors with normal vigor. They do not develop runt or graft-versus-host disease.

Although one might have expected to find by chance the simultaneous presence of both XX (female) and XY (male) cells in 50% of tetra-parental mice, only a very small proportion are hermaphrodites, the remainder being phenotypically normal males and females in approximately equal proportions, most of which are fertile. Dr. Beatrice Mintz has suggested that the paucity of intersexes may arise, at least in part, from competition and selection during early reproductive development.

Wegmann and his associates have reported that lymphocytes from tetraparental chimeras between the C3H and C57BL strains displayed cytotoxic activity *in vitro* against both C3H and C57BL fibroblasts from these strains and could react in mixed culture with lymphocytes from these strains. Furthermore, serum from the same donors could block this effect. No blocking was observed when sera from either of the parental strains or from (C3H × C57BL)F_1 hybrids was used. On the basis of these data the authors suggest that not all the potentially re-active lymphocytes of the donor lineage capable of reacting against the cellular antigens of the other zygote lineage and *vice versa* had been rendered tolerant or unresponsive.

It is pertinent to mention here that during the past few years the initial premise of Billingham, Brent, and Medawar that tolerance, as it applies to tissue allografts, represents a *central* failure of the immune response rather than peripheral interference of some kind between reac-tive lymphocytes and their targets, has been challenged. It has been pro-posed by some workers that tolerance, in reality, is due to the action of some kind of protective or "blocking" factor in serum that comes be-tween aggressive or "killer" lymphocytes and their specific target cells. Critical examination of the experimental evidence purporting to sustain this thesis reveals that there are grounds for belief that the degree of tolerance of skin allografts in the mice used as "tolerant subjects" may have been incomplete. Recent experiments by Beverley and her associates and by Dr. Leslie Brent and his co-workers have indicated that in mice in which an authentic and demonstrable degree of tolerance of skin allografts had been induced by neonatal inoculation of viable allogeneic lymphoid cells, there is a total lack of lymphoid cells capable of initiating any kind of graft-versus-host reactivity against donor cells or performing reactive roles in mixed leukocyte cultures *in vitro*. Furthermore the serum of such animals lacks the capacity to interfere with the activity of reactive cells *in vitro*.

Medawar has recently pointed out that tetraparental mice are, in an immunological sense, not necessarily equivalent to mice rendered tolerant by neonatal inoculation with lymphoid cells, which seem to be essential for the induction of complete and lasting tolerance in mice. Tetraparental mice are highly variable with regard to their level of chimerism in any particular tissue, and there is no easy means of assaying this.

It will be noted that in a genetic sense tetraparental mice are exact experimental counterparts of dispermic mosaic human beings since both represent the fusion products of two genetically dissimilar zygotes.

THE ENIGMA OF ARMADILLO QUADRUPLETS

The nine-banded armadillo, *Dasypus novemcinctus,* a resident of Texas, normally produces monozygotic quadruplets of similar sex. Cleavage of the initial zygote into four primordia occurs relatively late—after the formation of the amniotic vesicle. Each embryo has a specific zone of placenta that does not necessarily correspond to a morphologic quarter of the whole organ. However, dye injection experiments have failed to reveal the existence of vascular intercommunications between the placentas of individual embryos.

In 1962 Anderson and Benirschke reported that when skin grafts were exchanged between "identical" armadillo quadruplets—instead of behaving like autografts, or grafts exchanged between identical twins in man, a significant proportion incited either acute or chronic reactions on the part of their hosts to which some succumbed. This suggested that some kind of segregation of the genetic determinants of transplantation antigens must have occurred. The only other evidence of unequal inheritance in these one-egg quadruplets pertains to the patterns of the scutes in their bands. Clearly this puzzling phenomenon needs further investigation.

REFERENCES

Anderson, J. M., and Benirschke, K. 1963. "Fetal circulation in the placenta of *Dasypus novemcinctus,* linn. and their significance in transplantation." *Transplantation* 1:306–310.

Benirschke, K., and Brownhill, L. E. 1963. "Heterosexual cells in testes of chimeric marmoset monkeys." *Cytogenetics* 2:331–340.

Benirschke, K., and Driscoll, S. G. 1967. *The pathology of the human placenta.* Springer-Verlag, New York.

Beverley, P. C. L., Brent, L., Brooks, C., Medawar, P. B., and Simpson, E. 1973. "*In vitro* reactivity of lymphoid cells from tolerant mice." *Transpl. Proc.* 3:679–684.

Billingham, R. E., Lampkin, G. H., Medawar, P. B., and Williams, H. L. 1952. "Tolerance to homografts, twin diagnosis, and the freemartin condition in cattle." *Heredity* 6:201–212.

Brent, L., Brooks, C., Lubing, N., and Thomas, A. V. 1972. "Attempts to demonstrate an *in vivo* role for serum blocking factors in tolerant mice." *Transplantation* 14:382–378.

Burnet, F. M., and Fenner, F. 1949. *The production of antibodies.* McMillan, Melbourne.

Dunsford, I., Bowley, C. C., Hutchison, A. M., Thompson, J. S., Sanger, R., and Race, R. R. 1953. "A human blood-group chimera." *Brit. Med. J.* 2:81.

Hellström, K. E., and Hellström, I. 1972. "The role of serum factors ("blocking antibodies") as mediators of immunological non-reactivity to cellular antigens." In *Ontogeny of acquired immunity* (R. Porter and J. Knight, ed.). Ciba Foundation Symposium, Associated Scientific Publishers, Amsterdam, pp. 133–147.

Lillie, F. R. 1916. "The theory of the freemartin." *Science* 43:611–613.

Medawar, P. B. 1973. "Tolerance reconsidered—a critical survey." *Transpl. Proc.* 5:7–9.

Mintz, B., and Silvers, W. K. 1967. "Intrinsic immunological tolerance in allophenic mice." *Science* 158:1484–1487.

Ohno, S. 1967. "Sex chromosomes and sex-linked genes." In *Monographs on endocrinology,* Vol. 1 (A. Labhart, T. Mann, L. T. Samuels, and J. Zander, ed.). Springer-Verlag, New York, p. 192.

Owen, R. D. 1945. "Immunogenetic consequences of vascular anastomoses between bovine twins." *Science* 102:400–401.

Race, R. R., and Sanger, R. 1968. *Blood groups in man.* Blackwell, Oxford.

Stone, W. H., Friedman, J., and Fregin, A. 1964. "Possible somatic cell mating in twin cattle with erythrocyte mosaicism." *Proc. Nat. Acad. Sci.* 51:1036–1044.

Wegmann, T. G., Hellström, I., and Hellström, K. E. 1971. "Immunological tolerance: 'forbidden clones' allowed in tetraparental mice." *Proc. Nat. Acad. Sci.* 68:1644–1647.

Chapter 11

Maternal-Fetal Exchange of Cells and Its Consequences

Although anastomoses *never* develop between the blood circulations of mothers and their fetuses, even at the capillary level, placentas are not completely impermeable to the passage of cells across their trophoblastic frontier. Obviously on purely anatomic grounds the opportunity for exchange of cells is much greater in species with hemochorial placentas than in species in which the maternal and fetal circulations are more heavily 'insulated' from one another. For this reason and also because of the fact that natural transplacental passage or 'transplantation' of cells is responsible for several severe, immunologically based diseases that may affect perinatal infants, our knowledge of feto-maternal cellular exchanges in man surpasses that available for any other species.

Trophoblast Cells

In man, and certain other species including the chinchilla, from an early stage of gestation, multinucleate aggregates or sprouts of syncytiotrophoblast are continually breaking free, or being shed from, the placental villi and carried away in the maternal blood as it flows through the intervillous space. These trophoblastic fragments, exfoliated at the rate of about 100,000-200,000 per day from the twenty-sixth day of gestation onward in man, are highly susceptible to proteolytic enzymes *in vitro*. *In vivo* the majority probably undergo enzymatic degradation in the maternal blood stream. A small proportion are filtered out intact in the capillary bed of the lungs, however, where they gradually disappear unaccompanied by any local inflammatory or other host response. The apparent inability of these ectopic allografts of syncytiotrophoblast to proliferate and form benign metastases probably reflects their highly differentiated, end-cell status. Whether this normal physiologic process of feto-maternal deportation of trophoblast fragments has any functional significance is an unresolved question. Its possible immunologic significance will be discussed later. Deportation of trophoblast also occurs in

145

the opposite direction as evidenced by the presence of fragments in blood taken from the umbilical veins of fetuses at various stages of gestation or from the umbilical cord at the time of delivery.

BLOOD CELLS

It is now generally recognized that in man a small-scale, covert transplacental exchange of all the formed elements of blood, including platelets, is a common if not a normal event.

ERYTHROCYTES

Credit for the first direct demonstration of transplacental fetal-to-maternal passage of blood cells goes to Chown, who in 1954 showed by differential agglutination the presence of fetal Rh-positive erythrocytes in the blood of an Rh-negative mother. Since fetal-to-maternal passage of erythrocytes was first postulated as the cause of erythroblastosis fetalis or hemolytic disease of the newborn in 1938, many studies using different markers have confirmed that fetal erythrocytes can enter the maternal bloodstream from the eighth week of gestation onward. The incidence of this exchange in pregnant women increases with the length of gestation rising to about 30–40% in the third trimester. This suggests that either the integrity or efficiency of the placental barrier declines progressively as gestation progresses or the frequency of 'leakages,' (probably due to trivial, small-scale hemorrhages at the level of the trophoblastic villi) is simply a function of the aggregate area of maternal-fetal tissue interface in the placenta.

Labor and the delivery of the feto-placental unit further increase the chances of fetal erythrocytes entering the maternal circulation to 50%. Indeed, certain obstetrical maneuvers raise this figure above 85% as well as increase the volume of the cell traffic. Estimates have been made of the amount of blood a mother receives from her fetus by means of the acid elution technique of Kleihauer and Betke, which detects fetal erythrocytes in smears of maternal blood by virtue of their containing hemoglobin F (see Fig. 11-1). An effective sensitizing dosage is ½ cc or less of Rh incompatible blood in some individuals; however, much larger volumes are required in others. At this point in time there is no justification for the term, the "minimum sensitizing dose," which is sometimes used. It has been shown that 24–30% of postpartum patients whose blood smears contained fetal cells had received from 0.1–5.0 ml of fetal blood and that 1–2%, at least 50 ml.

Evidence is also accumulating that passage of maternal erythrocytes

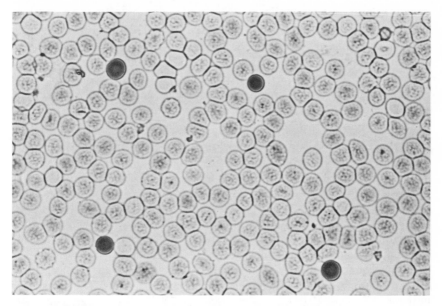

Fig. 11-1. Smear of venous blood from a woman taken during the ninth month of pregnancy and stained by the acid elution method of Kleihauer. This reveals the presence of four erythrocytes of fetal origin by virtue of the fact that they contain fetal hemoglobulin.

into the fetal circulation is probably a normal physiological event in humans. Indeed, massive amounts of blood are occasionally transferred, as for example in cases of neonatal plethora. There's little evidence bearing upon the incidence and extent of the cell traffic in this direction, however, that is not favored by the prevailing pressure differential.

LEUKOCYTES

It is inconceivable that an exchange of red cells could take place without accompanying leukocytes and platelets, though the tendency of the exchanged leukocytes to leave the host's bloodstream makes the detection and estimation of the magnitude of this exchange much more difficult; cytogenetic studies have revealed the presence of male (46XY) lymphocytes in the circulation of mothers who subsequently gave birth to male fetuses and there is evidence that lymphocytes of fetal origin sometimes persist in the circulation of the mothers for several weeks postpartum.

In 1969, Tuffrey and associates working at The Institute of Children's Health, University of London, London, presented cytogenetic evidence of a considerable maternal-to-fetal leukocytic traffic in mice. They mated female CBA strain mice that were homozygous for the T_6 chromosome marker with CBA (T_6T_6) males. Then, 2½ days later, they transferred fertilized eggs from the unrelated CFW strain of mice, which lack the T_6 marker, to the CBA females. The resulting litters comprised mice of the CBA and CFW strains, easily distinguishable by their coat colors. When they had grown up, the CFW animals were killed and various tissues including those of the lymphomyeloid complex were examined cytologically. According to these workers, 3–30% of alien (T_6T_6) labeled cells were identifiable among the dividing cells examined, indicative of a fairly high level of chimerism in some subjects. Although Tuffrey and her associates conceded that the CFW progeny might have acquired their "marked" cells from their CBA siblings *in utero,* they favored a maternal origin. In a subsequent study, using the same cytogenetic marker but an experimental design that excluded the possibility of complication by exchange of tagged cells between fetuses, chimerism attributable to transplacental passage of maternal cells proved to be quite infrequent. So far, attempts by other workers to confirm these interesting findings have been completely unsuccessful. The possibility remains, however, that for genetic reasons CFW mice gestated in CBA mothers may have been peculiarly susceptible to transplacental cellular exchange. Evidence will be presented below that this phenomenon does occur in rats, and maternal-to-fetal transmission of radioactively labeled leukocytes has been reported in the rabbit.

MALIGNANT CELLS

Instances of transmission of malignant disease from affected women to their fetuses are exceedingly rare. This is particularly surprising in the case of hematologic malignancies in which relatively large numbers of malignant stem cells may be present in the blood. It is pertinent to state that in the case of some nonhematologic tumors, including mammary carcinoma and osteosarcoma, malignant cells do gain access to and are disseminated in the patient's body by the vascular route. In an extensive review of the possible transmission of leukemia and allied diseases from mother to fetus, Drs. Diamondopoulous and Hertig found that among approximately 400 fetuses at risk transmission might have occurred in only 2 and possibly 4 more. Even here it is conceivable that the tumors in the progeny were initiated by an oncogenic agent rather than by a "cellular" graft or that by a rare coincidence both mother and offspring were afflicted independently by the same type of tumor.

Malignant melanoma is the only tumor which, unequivocally, can cross the placenta, probably after metastatic growth in this organ, and give rise to widespread metastases in the infant, usually resulting in death within a few months of delivery. At least six well-documented cases of this occurring are on record and in one of these complete regression of the tumor occurred in the infant. It is worth recalling (see Chapter 7) that choriocarcinoma of gestational origin is a tumor of fetal origin that consistently becomes established in the mother as a successful allograft but only rarely affects the fetus in whose trophoblastic tissue it originated.

These clinical observations afford no hint as to whether the very infrequent "success" of these tumor allografts of maternal origin can be attributed to induction of tolerance, to enhancement, or to chance genetic compatibility, especially at the HL-A complex. Evidence that the human fetus is immunocompetent long before birth (see Chapter 12) partially explains the extreme rarity of maternal-to-fetal transmission of tumors, though it affords no explanation for the unique success of the melanoma.

Red Cell Antigens:
Hemolytic Disease of the Newborn in Man

There are about 50 different erythrocyte isoantigens in man, determined by multiple alleles at different genetic loci, that can incite isoimmunization. Incompatibility for one or more of these antigens is a virtual certainty in all pregnancies. Fortunately these antigens vary widely with regard to their capacity to evoke clinically signficant levels of isoimmunization through pregnancy. In addition, their immunogenicity is influenced secondarily by compatibility or otherwise of the maternal environment with respect to the ABO blood group system.

Several prerequisites have to be satisfied before blood group incompatibility can jeopardize a fetus:

1. The fetus must have erythrocyte antigens that are not present on the mother's red blood cells.

2. Fetal erythrocytes bearing the incompatible antigen must gain access to the maternal circulation.

3. The mother must produce antibodies against the incompatible fetal erythrocyte antigens.

4. The antibodies produced by the mother must be capable of traversing the placenta (i.e., be of the IgG type so far as man is concerned) or otherwise gaining access to the infant's bloodstream.

5. Having gained access to the fetal circulation, these antibodies must combine with fetal cells bearing the antigen, leading to the removal of such cells from the circulation and their subsequent destruction.

RH ISOIMMUNIZATION

An erythrocyte antigen, called the *Rh antigen* or *rhesus factor* because of its initial discovery in the rhesus monkey, is present in 85% of all Caucasians. Approximately 93% of all Negroes and virtually all people of Mongolian origin possess this antigen. Most people, therefore, have this antigen; i.e., they are Rh-positive and cannot become sensitized to it through blood transfusion or pregnancy. Women who lack the antigen, i.e., are Rh-negative, may develop sensitivity to it through exposure to Rh-positive erythrocytes, however, as a result of receiving a blood transfusion or gestating an Rh-positive fetus.

Although, in fact, the Rh antigen is really a group of six antigens, C, D, E, and c, d, e, determined by pseudoallelic genes, nearly 99% of all cases of hemolytic disease of the newborn that are not caused by ABO blood group incompatibility are due to incompatibility with respect to the strong D antigen of the Rh blood group system. Persons are classified as Rh-positive or Rh-negative, respectively, on the presence or absence of the D antigen. Unlike the ABO determinants that are present on many types of cell, including leukocytes and epidermal cells, the distribution of Rh specificities is completely restricted to the plasma membranes of erythrocytes.

If red cells from an Rh-positive fetus enter the circulation of an Rh-negative mother, there are several possibilities. If the mother has not previously encountered the antigen, she may become sensitized and IgG antibodies will eventually appear in her serum. (see Fig. 11-2). There are now well-documented cases, however, in which (although no antibodies were detectable following primary stimulation) "anamnestic-type" responses occurred following secondary stimulation. In these situations it is quite possible that the initial small amount of D antigen that reaches antigen-sensitive cells is sufficient only to bring about proliferation of these cells with little differentiation into antibody-producing plasma cells. A second stimulus may lead to their further differentiation into antibody-producing cells.

A minimum of 0.1–0.5 ml of fetal blood is necessary to elicit sensitization. About 10% of all Rh-negative women fail to become sensitized, however, even after multiple Rh-positive pregnancies or through repeated injections of Rh-positive blood in the case of volunteers. Do such individuals who fail to become immunized following repeated exposure to D-positive erythrocytes represent adult tolerant subjects? It is possible, as suggested by Rowley and Fitch, that a very small amount of high-affinity antibody produced in response to a small antigenic stimulus could suppress the transformation of remaining antigen-sensitive cells

THE Rh NEGATIVE PROBLEM

FIRST PREGNANCY
Rh negative mother
Rh positive baby

SECOND PREGNANCY
Second Rh positive baby

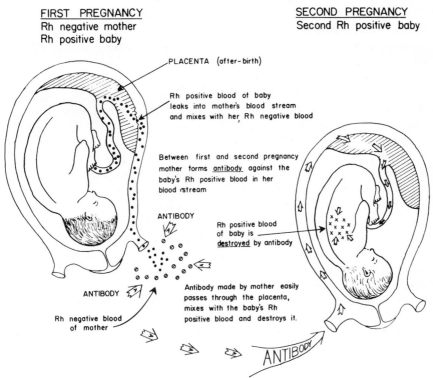

PLACENTA (after-birth)

Rh positive blood of baby leaks into mother's blood stream and mixes with her Rh negative blood

Between first and second pregnancy mother forms <u>antibody</u> against the baby's Rh positive blood in her blood stream

ANTIBODY

Rh positive blood of baby is <u>destroyed</u> by antibody

Antibody made by mother easily passes through the placenta, mixes with the baby's Rh positive blood and destroys it.

ANTIBODY

Rh negative blood of mother

ANTIBODY

Fig. 11-2. Illustrating how the natural passage or "leakage" of erythrocytes from the fetus across the placenta into its mother's bloodstream is responsible for erythroblastosis fetalis or Rh disease in some individuals. If the fetus is Rh-positive—e.g., has the Rh_0 D antigen on its erythrocytes—and the mother is Rh-negative—i.e., lacks this antigen—she will produce anti-D antibodies if Rh-positive blood enters her circulation. Transmission of these antibodies from her bloodstream to that of the fetus, across the placenta, will result in destruction of fetal erythrocytes and development of the disease. A similar disease results, though much more rarely, from fetal-maternal incompatibility with respect to other red cell antigens.

into antibody-forming cells and that this may be one way in which "true tolerance" to the D antigen occurs. Presumably this high-affinity antibody could compete successfully for further antigenic determinants introduced and lead to a state closely resembling tolerance.

Provided that a mother has had no previous exposure to the Rh antigen, the risk of her first Rh-positive infant being harmed is quite small; however, the hazard becomes progressively greater with each succeeding Rh-positive pregnancy. The effect of maternal isoimmunization on the Rh-positive fetus and newborn infant depends on the amount of Rh antibody that crosses the placenta. Attachment of the antibody to the fetal erythrocytes results in the rapid removal of these cells from the circulation, primarily by the spleen, and their subsequent destruction. The consequences include anemia, congestive heart failure, compensatory erythropoiesis, and hyperbilirubinemia, the last may result in the deposition of bilirubin in the brain, producing irreversible damage known as kernicterus.

There have been many ingenious attempts to explain the variation in response of Rh-negative persons exposed to Rh antigens. One interesting suggestion was that nonreactivity to Rh antigens might arise through gestation of Rh-negative fetuses in Rh-positive mothers, affording the offspring an opportunity to become tolerant of the antigens concerned. According to this theory an Rh-negative female child gestated in an Rh-positive mother should have an impaired capacity to form anti-D antibodies when, in adult life, she bears an Rh-positive fetus, in comparison with an Rh-negative female gestated by an Rh-negative mother. No factual support has been forthcoming for this attractive idea. Indeed, rarely, Rh-negative females actually receive their first sensitizing dose of Rh-positive cells *in utero* from their *mothers*. These individuals may comprise from 1–2% of all Rh-sensitized patients and usually manifest as "first-pregnancy Rh isoimmunization."

A nonspecific weakening of the faculty of immunologic reactivity during pregnancy has also been invoked to help account for the variation in response of Rh-negative persons to the Rh antigens. Again this idea lacks factual support.

The most likely explanation for the low frequency of sensitization during the first pregnancy at risk turns upon the behavior of the Rh-incompatible but ABO-compatible erythrocytes in the maternal environment. The life-span of such cells is *long*—100 to 200 days. The earliest that Rh isoimmunization has ever been detected in a pregnant subject is 24 weeks of pregnancy. ABO-compatible, Rh-incompatible erythrocytes in an Rh-negative mother seem to be well tolerated and do not become immunogenic until they are near the end of their life-span and "tagged" for clearance by the maternal spleen where the foreign Rh antigens are recognized by antigen-sensitive cells in the host's lymphoid centers.

The risk of subsequent sensitization of Rh-negative mothers bearing Rh-positive fetuses is now known to depend on

1. The magnitude of the transplacental hemorrhage of Rh-incompatible blood.

2. The specific Rh genotype of the fetus. There are approximately 12,000 D-antigen sites on the membrane of a D-positive erythrocyte. With the aid of ^{131}I-labeled anti-D antibody it has been confirmed that cDE cells react more strongly than CDe cells and that cDE/cDE cells

agglutinate more strongly than any other cells with respect to the Rh system. The presence of C in the genome decreases the number of D antigenic determinants available for binding with the labeled immuno-globulin and probably reduces the immunogenicity of such a cell.

ABO blood group incompatibility between mother and fetus has been shown to afford an interesting natural protective mechanism against the risk of Rh sensitization. It has been shown that the risk of immunizing a mother by an ABO-incompatible Rh-positive pregnancy is approximately 20% that of an ABO-compatible Rh-positive pregnancy. Its *modus operandi* is illustrated by the following example. If a group O, Rh-negative mother gestates a group A, Rh-positive fetus, fetal erythrocytes entering her circulation will undergo lysis or opsonization by the naturally occurring anti-A antibodies in her serum, resulting in removal of these cells in the liver by processes that are unlikely to result in sensitization. Findings of Drs. J. C. Woodrow and W. T. A. Donohoe indicate that anti-D antibodies are eight times more likely to appear in the postnatal period following first pregnancies that are ABO-compatible than when the first pregnancy is ABO-incompatible. Recognition of this natural protection against the risk of hemolytic disease of the newborn, by Dr. Philip Levine in 1958, stimulated the intensive research that eventually resulted in the deliberate administration of anti-Rh immuno-globulin as a successful means of preventing primary Rh isoimmunization in patients at risk (see below).

Three procedures are available for treatment of hemolytic disease of the newborn, either prior to delivery to help assure that the infant will be viable at birth or after delivery to increase the likelihood that the live-born infant will survive. Briefly these are

1. Induction of labor prematurely if there is evidence (e.g., results of spectrophotometric analysis of amniotic fluid obtained by amnio-centesis) that the fetus will not survive until term or will be so severely affected at birth that even exchange transfusion may be unable to save its life.

2. Exchange transfusion that is performed in the first few hours of life and has saved thousands of lives since it was introduced in 1946 (see Table 11-1). Its principal goal is removal of target erythrocytes, which, if destroyed, would have raised the level of serum bilirubin, and their replacement with group O, Rh-negative fresh red cells that will enjoy a normal survival time in the infant.

3. Intrauterine transfusions of compatible blood may be given in cases in which analysis of amniotic fluid indicates that the fetus is in danger of dying within a few weeks and is too immature to survive premature delivery. Packed Rh-negative erythrocytes rather than whole blood are used and they are introduced into the peritoneal cavity of the fetus.

Table 11-1

Criteria for exchange blood transfusion of affected infant of
RH-sensitized mother

1. A hemoglobin level of 14 g/100 ml or below in infant. Normal value is 2× this level.

2. Rapid rise of bilirubin in the infant's blood.

3. If the cord bilirubin level is above 4.5 mg/100 ml, an exchange transfusion is done immediately after birth.

4. A level of serum bilirubin of 20 mg/100 ml in the first few days of life is used as an absolute indication for exchange transfusion.

They are gradually absorbed from this site into its bloodstream via the draining lymphatic vessels. Usually several intrauterine transfusions are given at spaced intervals followed by early delivery and exchange blood transfusion immediately afterward.

Rh Prophylaxis:
Circumvention of Maternal Sensitization

The principle of the procedure employed to prevent Rh-negative women from becoming sensitized to Rh-positive blood was discovered by Theobald Smith in 1909. He showed that diphtheria toxin can be rendered nonantigenic if it is administered to an animal simultaneously with large amounts of the specific antitoxin. Other workers have confirmed this and demonstrated that the phenomenon that it illustrates applies to many other antigen-antibody systems.

In 1961, Dr. R. Finn and his colleagues, mindful of the protective role of ABO incompatibility against Rh sensitization, made the ingenious proposal that similar protection might be afforded artificially by passive immunization of subjects at risk with anti-D antibody. His experimental studies established the feasibility of this idea. Simultaneously, though quite independently, Drs. Freda, Gorman, and Pollack, exploring the application of the "Theobold Smith principle," established that administration of excess anti-D antibody to Rh-negative male volunteers after a normally effective sensitizing dose of Rh-positive erythrocytes prevented primary immunization. Pertinent to this line of inquiry were previous observations of other workers that group O, Rh-positive cells treated *in vitro* with anti-D antibody failed to immunize group O, Rh-negative male volunteers and that coating the red cells with anti-D antibody *in vitro* caused them to undergo rapid clearance from the host's circulation after they had been administered.

Large-scale clinical trials on the influence of injecting Rh-negative women with anti-D antibody soon after parturition have given highly encouraging results. Thousands of treated patients have been followed for a 6-month period postinjection following one or multiple Rh-incompatible pregnancies. The failure rates in the United States following one incompatible pregnancy in which passive immunization was given are of the order of 0.5%. The cumulative incidence of antibodies appearing in the interval following a second Rh-incompatible but treated pregnancy is 2%. It is of interest that the highest failure rate in treated mothers occurs in individuals that demonstrate only very few Rh-positive fetal cells in their circulation following their delivery. Where large amounts of Rh-positive fetal blood are found in the maternal circulation after delivery of the first child, it is likely that fetal-to-maternal hemorrhage was a late event in pregnancy. In this circumstance it can be expected that immunization will be successfully suppressed by passive antibody. By far the most cogent evidence of the efficacy of this procedure is its proved ability to protect Rh-negative mothers through *multiple* Rh-incompatible pregnancies.

CURRENT VIEWS ON MECHANISMS OF SUPPRESSION OF THE IMMUNE RESPONSE TO ERYTHROCYTE ANTIGENS BY ANTIBODY

In recent years, since the pioneering studies of Uhr and Bauman, there have been extensive studies highlighting the physiological role of antibody in the induction and control of the immune response. There are certain facts worth enumerating that have emerged recently relating to antibody-mediated immunosuppression:

1. Both *in vivo* and *in vitro* studies show that the suppressive effect of antibody is antigen-specific.

2. The stronger the antigen, i.e., the greater the number of antigenic sites represented on or in the plasma membranes of the cell, the more difficult it is to suppress the primary immune response.

3. The longer the interval between the introduction of the foreign antigen and the administration of the specific antibody, the less likely it is that suppression will be achieved.

4. Active immunosuppression requires a considerable amount of antibody, i.e., antibody excess. Mollison and Hughes-Jones demonstrated that clearance of 99% of the antigen was achieved when 10% of the antigen sites were occupied by specific antibody. In Rh-negative women, 10 μg

of anti-D antibody will suppress immunity following the injection of 1 ml of Rh-positive erythrocytes.

5. The secondary immune response cannot be altered by specific passive antibody.

6. Antigen excess in the presence of high-affinity specific antibody leads to potentiation or enhancement of the immune response.

By what means can specific high-affinity antibody avert the appropriate contact of foreign antigenic determinants with "helper" cells to prevent the proliferation and differentiation of antibody-producing cells? Three possible ways by which antibody may interfere with the elicitation of immunity are

1. By its blocking or masking of foreign antigenic sites so that antigen in appropriate immunogenic form never appears or incites an immune response in lymphoid centers,

2. By blocking or binding antigenic determinants either within or on the surface of macrophages so that effective contact with antigen-sensitive cells is prevented,

3. By a direct suppressive or inhibitory activity on specific antigen-sensitive cells themselves.

There is presently solid experimental evidence that specific antibody can and does act in all of the ways above. Ryder and Schwartz showed that specific antibodies can act on macrophages in such a way as to inhibit their ability to transmit foreign antigenic determinants once processed to antigen-sensitive cells. Rowley and Fitch showed that specific antibody bound to immunocompetent spleen cells rendered them unresponsive when subsequently confronted with the antigen.

Thus it appears that in instances where immunosuppression is achieved, the following criteria are met: First, specific, high-affinity antibody binds within or on the surface of macrophages, preventing optimal access of free antigenic determinants to receptor sites on antigen-sensitive cells. Second, antigen, once altered by specific antibody, is in some instances processed or cleared in areas of the lymphomyeloid complex deficient in antigen-sensitive cells.

ABO BLOOD GROUP INCOMPATIBILITY AS A CAUSE OF HEMOLYTIC DISEASE OF THE PERINATAL SUBJECT

Although ABO blood group incompatible pregnancies are much more common than Rh-incompatible pregnancies, hemolytic disease of the newborn secondary to ABO incompatibility presents a minor clinical problem since only a small proportion of ABO incompatible pregnancies result in damage to the erythrocytes of the fetuses or newborn. These disease-associated pregnancies are largely confined to type A or B infants gestated by type O mothers. Even when the disease does occur, it is less severe than when it follows an Rh-incompatible maternal-fetal relationship.

Although the pathophysiology of hemolytic disease of the newborn due to ABO incompatibility is closely similar to that due to Rh incompatibility, there are important basic immunologic differences between the two situations. Unlike the situation with Rh antigens, substances having antigenic determinants closely similar to the A and B blood group substances are widely distributed in the environment, being present in certain plant materials and foodstuffs. Thus, during infancy, individuals develop antibodies—the so-called "natural" isoagglutinins—to ABO incompatible erythrocytes as a consequence of a natural covert sensitization. More pertinent for us is the fact that prior to their first pregnancy, blood group A women already have antibodies to type B erythrocytes and, conversely, type B women have antibodies to type A red cells and, of course, type O women have antibodies to both A and B red cells. Fortunately, in blood group A and B individuals, these natural isoagglutinins are usually of the IgM (19S macroglobulin) class, which are unable to cross the placenta and so harm potentially susceptible fetuses. In type O individuals, however, the antibodies generated by natural exposure to A and B blood group substances belong to both IgM and the IgG (7S) classes, and the latter can cross the placenta and cause hemolytic disease.

Unlike the situation with Rh incompatibility, 40–50% of cases of hemolytic disease caused by ABO group incompatibility are *first-born* infants. For unknown reasons, siblings following an infant affected by ABO hemolytic disease are less likely to develop clinically significant hemolytic disease, despite their possession of the same "offending" red cell antigen.

Although feto-maternal incompatibility for minor blood group antigens can also cause hemolytic disease of the perinate, it is rare, accounting for only 1–2% of all cases of hemolytic disease of the newborn. The Kell and Kidd blood groups are those most frequently involved and, less frequently, the MNS and Duffy groups.

MATERNAL LEUKOCYTE ISOIMMUNIZATION AND ITS CONSEQUENCES

The formation of isoagglutinins to leukocytes after multiple transfusions has been well-documented and subsequent work by Drs. Rose Payne and M. B. Rolfs in the United States and by Dr. Jan van Rood in Holland established that in man leukocyte agglutinins may appear in the maternal serum following multiple pregnancies. According to Dr. Payne, these antibodies are present in the sera of about 25% of women who have had more than three pregnancies. These findings afford additional evidence of both the occurrence and the incidence of fetal-maternal transmission of leukocytes since the antigens concerned are not present on erythrocytes. Furthermore, their presence on trophoblast in an effective form remains uncertain (see Chapter 6). Since multiparous women can only form antibodies against the leukocyte antigens transmitted to their fetuses by their husbands and absent in themselves, their antibodies are necessarily of limited specificity, sometimes being capable of recognizing a single antigen. Such individuals are an invaluable source of sera for histocompatibility testing since most of the serologically detectable antigenic determinants, referred to as "leukocyte antigens" are in fact histocompatibility antigens. These isoantibodies persist at relatively high titers in the sera of multiparous women for many years after their last pregnancy.

Although transplacental passage of these leukocyte antibodies from mother to fetus has been demonstrated, few of the infants born of leukocyte-sensitized mothers have manifested clinical evidence of any damaging influence of the antibodies concerned. There are some case reports, however, associating abnormal susceptibility to infection during the first month or two of life with leukopenia and the presence of these antibodies.

In a retrospective study reported in 1970, Dr. Paul Terasaki and his associates obtained suggestive data that women with HL-A (human leukocyte antigen) antibodies give birth to a significantly higher proportion of infants with congenital anomalies than women without these antibodies. These investigators postulated that antibodies produced by mothers against the HL-A antigens of fetuses have an adverse effect on fetuses in subsequent pregnancies.

Isoimmunization of mothers to platelet antigens through blood transfusions or natural transplacental "transfusion" with fetal platelets during pregnancy may also occur. The antiplatelet antibodies produced by these perfectly normal mothers readily cross the placenta and may destroy fetal platelets, predisposing the fetus to severe hemorrhage especially during the trauma associated with birth. There is also an autoimmune disease known as idiopathic thrombocytopenic purpura (ITP) characterized by a deficiency in platelets and increased capillary fragility. Pregnancy in women suffering from this disease results in a transient platelet deficiency in the infants as a consequence of transfer of the autoantibodies concerned across the placenta.

In mice, too, antibodies detectable as isohemagglutinins, and corresponding to histocompatibility determinants inherited by fetuses from their fathers, appear in the sera of multiparous females. The observation that repeated matings of sterile females with unrelated males fails to incite the formation of these antibodies indicates that the conceptuses rather than seminal products must be the source of the antigenic stimulus.

THE PHENOMENON OF ALLOTYPE SUPPRESSION

It is appropriate to consider the phenomenon of allotype suppression at this point since although no cellular interchanges between mother and fetuses are involved, some of the key events are analogous to those we have just been considering. Immunoglobulins have genetically determined antigenic markers known as allotypes, which, like blood group and transplantation antigens, are inherited in a simple Mendelian manner. The quantity of a particular class of immunoglobulin in the serum bearing a particular allotypic specificity can easily be determined. It has been shown that rabbits that lack a particular allotype can usually be immunized against it and females immunized against their mate's allotype can transmit to their fetuses antibodies that are specific for a paternally inherited fetal immunoglobulin allotype.

The effect of this maternal-fetal transmission of antibodies to a fetal allotype is to suppress production of immunoglobulins bearing the marker allotype, and this is compensated for by an increase in the concentration of an immunoglobulin allotype determined by a maternally inherited allelic gene.

For example, in heterozygous B^1/B^2 offspring of B^1/B^1 mothers immunized with their mate's B^2 immunoglobulin, there is suppression of immunoglobulin with the B^2 marker and a compensatory increase in B^1 allotype immunoglobulins, so that the overall concentration of IgG in affected animals is normal.

Although the maternally transmitted antibodies causing the phenotypic suppression only persist in the infant rabbit's circulation for a few weeks, the allotypic suppression may persist throughout the animal's life. The suppressed allotype usually appears eventually, however, gradually increasing in concentration. This effect of allotype suppression and compensatory allotypic expression reflects the operation of a mechanism that regulates the relative concentrations of immunoglobulins synthesized by the various immunoglobulin genes. Immunocompetent B lymphocytes have allotypic specificities on their surfaces and it is believed that the anti-allotype antibodies interact with the antigen at the cell surface, resulting either in the destruction of those cells committed to synthesize a particular allotype of immunoglobulin or blocking of their capacity to differentiate in one direction but allowing them to synthesize an alternative allotype.

Allotype suppression by specific antibodies also occurs in heterozygous mice as a consequence of their prenatal and/or postnatal exposure to maternal antibody. In this species the suppression observed is less complete and of shorter duration than in the rabbit in the absence of continued antiallotype treatment. It has been claimed that both maternal and fetal deaths occur in pregnant mice having alloantibodies directed against paternal immunoglobulin types. For example, following immunization of BALB/c females with immunoglobulin from C57BL/6 donors and subsequent mating with males of this strain, there was a considerable reduction in the number of surviving progeny and almost 50% of the females succumbed at term. When the experiment was performed with C57 females and BALB/c males, the pregnant females survived but failed to deliver live offspring. These interesting findings urgently need confirmation.

In man, the possibility exists that the receipt of a genetically appropriate blood transfusion by a woman might, by chance, lead to immunization against certain allotypes of her husband, which might have serious consequences during a subsequent pregnancy.

PARITY-INDUCED ALTERATIONS IN MATERNAL REACTIVITY TO ALLOGRAFTS

The various findings so far described indicate, first, that cells from fetuses of certain species, notably man, do gain access to the maternal circulation and probably by the regional lymph nodes draining the uterus since these enlarge during heterospecific pregnancies. Second, the mother is immunologically aware of, and is indeed stimulated by, some of the alien antigens of her fetus.

Long before maternal hemagglutinin responses to fetal transplantation antigens were discovered, grafting experiments employing test tumor or skin allografts, from either the offspring, its father, or a member of the paternal inbred strain, were performed to determine whether heterospecific pregnancies could alter the mother's reactivity to the tissue antigens concerned. In cattle, but not in sheep, suggestive evidence has been obtained that pregnancy sometimes results in sensitization of the dam in respect of her offspring's antigens. In women there is some rather equivocal evidence that habitual spontaneous abortion may be associated with the development of sensitivity to paternal transplantation antigens.

In mice, careful studies have failed to produce any evidence that heterospecific pregnancies ever lead to *curtailment* of the life expectancy of skin allografts from the paternal strain, i.e., to sensitization. On the contrary, exactly the opposite may occur, leading to a long-lasting specific weakening of a female's capacity to reject paternal strain skin allografts. If tumor allografts rather than skin allografts are used to test the females' reactivity, more impressive prolongations of graft survival are obtained on account of their superior capacity to override minor degrees of immunological opposition. The extent of this parity-induced "tolerance" or specific impairment of reactivity has been shown to depend on (1) the magnitude of the genetic disparity between the parents, being most impressive when major histocompatibility locus differences are excluded and (2) the parity of the female. Host reactivity decreases with parity up to a certain point, but only when relatively weak antigens are involved, such as the H-Y factor in C57BL/6 mice, is it completely abolished. Studies by Drs. Edward J. Breyere and S. O. Burhoe at American University in Washington indicate that the incompleteness of parity-induced tolerance probably reflects the induction of complete and lasting tolerance to some paternal strain antigens and unchanged or only partially suppressed reactivity to others—probably the more important or stronger antigenic determinants involved. Indeed, some of these antigenic determinants may not be expressed by the fetal cells that gain access to the pregnant females.

That the antigenic stimulus responsible for inducing the maternal unresponsiveness or tolerance originates from the *fetus* before parturition is indicated by observations made by Drs. Porter and Breyere. These investigators first showed that interstrain matings of strain BALB/c female mice, whose uterine horns had been ligated or whose ovaries had been transplanted subcutaneously (to preclude pregnancy but preserve their normal ovarian endocrine status), with DBA/2 males failed to weaken their reactivity to DBA/2 test grafts. Second, they demonstrated that despite excision of the gravid uterine horns near term from BALB/c females pregnant by DBA/2 males, evidence of impaired reactivity was still obtained.

On the basis of the various observations that multiparity in mice resulting from matings with males of an unrelated strain leads to both isoantibody formation and specific weakening of reactivity to allografts of skin and sarcomas (but heightened reactivity to leukemic test grafts, when the male and female differ at the major H-2 locus) Drs. Kaliss and Dagg of the Jackson Laboratory, Bar Harbor, suggested that immunological enhancement rather than immunological tolerance might be the principle underlying this parity-induced weakening of allograft reactivity. The heightened reactivity of the multiparous mice to leukemic test grafts and, indeed, to normal cells of the lymphomyeloid complex was reasonably attributed to the well-known vulnerability of these cells to the complement-dependent cytotoxic action of humoral antibodies.

Initial shortcomings of this enhancement hypothesis were, first, inability to produce enhancement in normal mice by transfer of serum from multiparous donors of the same strain and, second, the absence of any correlation between the presence or absence of hemagglutinins in the multiparous females and their reactivity to sarcoma test allografts. Kaliss and Dagg did not attach great significance to the latter since the antibodies responsible for the enhancing activity probably differed qualitatively from those responsible for the hemagglutinating activity. Subsequent findings have done much to strengthen the attraction of this theory. It has been shown that there are marked cyclical undulations in the titers of isoagglutinins induced by multiparity which were not associated with the stage of pregnancy and which occurred in females that were not pregnant at the time of testing. Furthermore, there was no evidence of any "anamnestic response" following a successive heterospecific pregnancy. The observation that pregnancy-induced hemagglutinins have a very short half-life after passive transfer is also relevant here.

Dr. Graham Currie of The Chester Beatty Research Institute in England has carried out a well-controlled investigation in which strain A_2G female mice were mated with CBA strain males and cells of a chemically induced CBA sarcoma were used as test allografts to detect altered immunological reactivity. He was able to demonstrate a feeble though definite degree of specific impairment of reactivity to paternal tissue antigens early in the first interstrain pregnancy. More important is his observation that the capacity of virgin A_2G females to destroy grafts of the tumor was significantly impaired by repeated inoculations of serum from A_2G females multiparous by CBA males. On the basis of these findings the conclusion was drawn that immunological enhancement is the mechanism responsible for the pregnancy-induced specific unresponsiveness to paternal antigens.

In the mouse Breyere and Spiess have recently shown that repeated pregnancies of BALB/c female mice by allogeneic (but H-2 locus compatible) DBA/2 males specifically weaken a *preexisting* immunity to DBA/2 tumor allografts. The females were immunized by a single subcutaneous injection of DBA blood followed 10 days later by an inoculation of tumor cells. When subsequently challenged with a tumor cell graft it grew progressively in a significantly higher percentage of multiparous females than in immunized control virgin mice of similar age. This weakening of host reactivity increased with multiparity, but only up to a point. Four pregnancies resulted in the maximal effect obtainable, which enabled tumors to grow in about 70% of the mice. Alternately mating and challenging mice with the tumor graft did not weaken their initial resistance.

In C57BL/6 mice, five to seven pregnancies by syngeneic males renders the majority of the females completely incapable of rejecting grafts of skin from adult C57 male donors, and eight or more pregnancies totally abolish reactivity to the Y antigen in all females. These unresponsive females are not demonstrably chimeric, and various observations, including Jeekel's finding that this unresponsiveness is transferable to virgin females by means of serum, indicate that enhancement is the underlying phenomenon. Some previous analyses of this seemingly simplest of all possible examples of pregnancy-induced unresponsiveness involved mating normal females with sterile males, or sterile females with normal males. These revealed that mere inoculation of spermatozoa or seminal fluid sufficed to induce unresponsiveness. The important findings that the Y antigen does not express itself until *after* birth and sexual maturation and that castration of newborn males prevents its appearance make it seem very unlikely that the stimulus for this particular parity-induced unresponsiveness is transplacental leakage into the mother of cells or other material from her male fetuses. A systemic influence of repeated antigenic stimulation of the female reproductive tract through mating affords a reasonable explanation.

CONSEQUENCES OF FETAL EXPOSURE TO MATERNAL CELLS

Maternally Induced Tolerance

Ever since the principle of immunological tolerance was first worked out with tissue transplantation antigen systems in very young animals, the possibility has been entertained that offspring might "naturally" become tolerant of their mother's tissue antigens (i.e., those whose genetic determinants they had failed to inherit) as a consequence of exposure in fetal life to maternal cells (obviously leukocytes are the most likely candidates). Studies have been undertaken to explore this possibility in mice, rabbits, guinea pigs, cattle, sheep, and man but the results, in general, have been very disappointing. Where outbred animals had to be used, survival times of paternal and maternal skin allografts on their progeny were compared; but when inbred strains were available, experiments of more sophisticated design and capable of revealing feebler degrees of maternally induced tolerance were possible.

Because of its long gestation period (about 60 days) and its hemochorial type of placenta, the guinea pig seemed to be a favorable subject for investigating this phenomenon. Billingham and Silvers reciprocally backcrossed F_1 hybrid progeny of the inbred strains No. 2 and No. 13 to strain No. 13 to produce two similar, genetically defined but heterogeneous populations of animals that differed only insofar as one group of animals had been gestated in an F_1 hybrid maternal milieu, affording them an opportunity to incorporate F_1 cells bearing strain No. 2 antigens prenatally. To test for any alteration of immunological reactivity this might have caused, both groups of R_2 progeny were challenged, when they were 30 days old, with skin allografts from strain No. 2 donors. The survival time distributions of the two series of grafts were closely similar, indicating that maternally induced tolerance must be a very rare phenomenon in the guinea pig if it occurs at all. A similar conclusion had previously been reached from an experiment of similar design conducted upon mice of strains A and CBA. Dr. Barbara Sanford, using tumors as test grafts, obtained evidence of increased susceptibility of backcross progeny gestated in F_1 hybrid female mice, however, which was suggestive of maternally induced tolerance.

Two other approaches to find out whether maternally induced tolerance occurs must be mentioned. Drs. Jones and P. L. Krohn of the University of Birmingham, England, took A strain female mice that had been rendered tolerant of CBA tissue antigens by neonatal intravenous inoculation of CBA cells and replaced their ovaries by functional ovarian grafts from CBA donors. These females were mated with CBA males so that the resultant CBA fetuses were gestated from conception onward in an A strain maternal environment, affording them ample opportunity to receive A strain cells transplacentally. None of these animals proved to be tolerant of CBA test skin allografts. Billingham, Palm, and Silvers carried out an essentially similar experiment in rats of the Ag-B locus incompatible Lewis and BN strains. They took (BN × Lewis) F_1 hybrid females, replaced their ovaries with those from Lewis females, and subsequently mated them with males of the Lewis strain. Lewis fetuses were thereby caused to be gestated in an F_1 hybrid milieu, thus exposing them to BN antigens. When they were 3 days old, the offspring were challenged with BN skin allografts—a procedure that had previously been shown to reveal weak, transient degrees of tolerance that would have escaped detection if test grafting had been delayed until the animals had grown up. None of these animals gave evidence of being tolerant. Indeed, some of them rejected their test skin allografts more rapidly than Lewis infants gestated by Lewis mothers, suggesting that they had been specifically presensitized. This sensitivity might have resulted from exposure to a very low dosage of maternal cells at the time of parturition.

In the rabbit there is a report of a slight but significant prolongation of survival of maternal as compared with paternal skin grafts on newborn progeny in a situation in which the parents were fairly closely related. If the test grafting operation was delayed until 3 days after birth, however, the difference in survival times became marginal. When greater genetic disparities between the parents were involved, grafts from the mothers enjoyed no advantage over those from the fathers. Indeed there was suggestive evidence that some of the offspring had been sensitized to maternal antigens.

Neither in cattle nor in sheep have appropriate grafting tests yielded any evidence of maternally induced tolerance. In man a claim made by Dr. Lyndon Peer and his associates in 1960 that children sometimes accept skin allografts from their mothers for much longer than from their fathers has never been confirmed, although the present authors are aware of unpublished attempts to do so. Certainly no evidence has been forthcoming that renal allografts from maternal donors are more successful than from paternal donors as one would have expected from Peer's findings.

Obviously, maternally induced tolerance of tissue antigens is a rare phenomenon if it occurs at all, possibly because too few maternal cells gain access to the fetuses. In part, this may be a consequence of the unfavorable blood pressure gradient—i.e., the blood pressure in the fetal placenta exceeding that of the maternal intervillous space.

ATTEMPTS TO AUGMENT THE TRANSPLACENTAL EXCHANGE OF CELLS

Several attempts have been made to increase the magnitude of the transplacental cellular traffic between mother and fetus and so increase the likelihood of procuring maternally induced tolerance in the fetus. In 1957, Dr. Alena Lengerová, of the Czechoslovak Academy of Sciences, ingeniously irradiated the exteriorized gravid uterine horns of outbred female rats on the fifteenth day of pregnancy, shielding the body of the mother. When the 4-week-old progeny were challenged with grafts of maternal skin, the majority accepted these for more than 200 days. Grafts from mothers to unirradiated offspring, or from unrelated females to previously irradiated hosts, were all rejected within 30 days. This interesting finding was attributed to irradiation-facilitated maternal induction of tolerance. Subsequently, Drs. H. Ramseier and R. L. Brent, working in Philadelphia, locally irradiated the placentas of (DA × Lewis) F_2 hybrid rat fetuses of 15 days' gestation in the uteri of (DA × Lewis) F_1 mothers previously mated with (DA × Lewis) F_1 males. Following weaning, each survivor received a DA strain skin allograft and a Lewis strain skin allograft. Control data were afforded by similarly test grafting F_2 hybrid rats whose placentas had not been irradiated. The life expectancy of the DA grafts on the irradiated F_2 population was superior to that of similar grafts on the unirradiated controls, supporting the premise that local irradiation of the placentas had indeed increased the maternal $\longrightarrow$ fetal cellular traffic, resulting in tolerance in those instances where the genetic disparity between mother and fetus was not too great. The experimental results were asymmetrical, however, in that no evidence was obtained of maternally induced tolerance to Lewis tissue antigens.

Two groups of investigators, working independently, have reported that administration of hyaluronidase and/or histamine to pregnant outbred rabbits partially or completely abbrogated the ability of a significant proportion of their progeny to reject grafts of maternal skin. Indeed, Drs. Najarian and Dixon found that many of their does behaved as if they were partially or even completely tolerant of their offspring's skin. Furthermore it was shown that hyaluronidase treatment increased the number of maternal erythrocytes that normally crossed the placenta during the last 2 weeks of pregnancy by a factor of 2.

In 1965 Dr. Peter Stastny, working at the University of Texas Southwestern Medical School at Dallas, reported that Sprague-Dawley female rats, mated with males of the same outbred stock and grafted with skin from Lewis strain donors when they were pregnant, gave birth to young that reacted to subsequent allografts of Lewis skin just as if they themselves had been sensitized. Since transplantation immunity to skin allografts normally is only transferable by means of living cells of the lymphocytic series and not by putatively immune serum, these and other observations that Dr. Stastny reported raised the interesting but remote (in the light of the evidence reviewed above) possibility that alteration in the maternal immunologic status might have resulted in compromise of the placental barrier by "activated" maternal cells. The present authors subsequently confirmed Stastny's findings, first with the same rat stocks he'd used and subsequently with inbred Fischer rats exposed to alloantigens from Lewis strain donors.

In the course of our analysis of this phenomenon, virgin Fischer females were mated with Fischer males. Then, at various stages of gestation the females received a single intraperitoneal injection of a suspension of 100×10^6 viable Lewis strain lymphoid cells. The Fischer progeny were challenged with skin allografts from Lewis donors 21 days after birth. The survival times of these grafts indicated that the capacity of many of their hosts to react against Lewis tissue antigens had been significantly *weakened* as a consequence of the inoculation of their mothers with Lewis cells 5-7 days before, or even only a few *hours* before their birth. Inoculation of the mothers *after* parturition had no influence on the subsequent immunologic status of the sucklings *vis à vis* Lewis antigens. The finding that, in these experiments, unresponsiveness rather than immunity was usually the outcome probably reflected the known high degree of tolerance-responsiveness of infant Fischer rats to Lewis cellular antigens. For example, intravenous injection of as few as 250,000 Lewis bone marrow cells into neonatal Fischer rats will induce a high degree of tolerance of Lewis skin allografts in 90% of them.

Encouraged by these findings, and using the same rat strain combination, we brought another experimental approach to bear on the problem of maternally induced tolerance (see Fig. 11-3). Sexually mature virgin female Fischer strain rats were treated with an immunosuppressant drug, *cyclophosphamide,* or *Cytoxan,* to destroy their lymphoid and bone marrow tis-

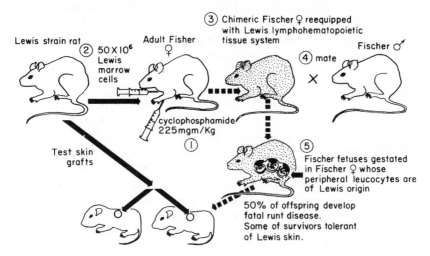

Fig. 11-3. Illustrating the design of an experiment to demonstrate the possible induction of tolerance of maternal tissue alloantigens, which the progeny have not inherited, as a consequence of transplacental leakage of maternal leukocytes. Young, virgin Fischer rats were treated with a cytotoxic drug, cyclophosphamide, to destroy their lymphohematopoietic tissue system and rehabilitated by infusing living bone marrow cells from Lewis strain donors. This resulted in the virtually total replacement of the host's bone marrow, lymphoid tissue, and peripheral blood leukocytes with similar cells of Lewis type. After the rats had recovered from this preparative treatment, they were mated with Fischer males in the hope that normal placental permeability to cells would allow sufficient Lewis leukocytes to enter the developing Fischer fetuses to induce tolerance of Lewis tissue antigens. Despite their healthy appearance at birth, about 50% of the progeny developed and succumbed to runt or graft-versus-host disease by the twenty-fifth day postpartum. When they were 20 days old, the healthy survivors were challenged with skin allografts from Lewis donors. Prolonged survival of many of these grafts afforded evidence of maternally induced tolerance.

sues—a potentially lethal procedure; 24 hours later these animals received a "lifesaving" transfusion of bone marrow cells from adult rats of the unrelated Lewis strain. As Drs. George Santos and Albert Owens of John Hopkins University School of Medicine had previously shown, this procedure results in complete replacement of the host's bone marrow, lymphoid tissue, and blood leukocytes by cells of graft origin—i.e., they become chimeras and, as one would expect, are completely tolerant of grafts of Lewis skin.

After these Fischer rats had recovered from replacement of their "lymphohematopoietic" tissue system by one of Lewis origin, they were mated with Fischer males. The resultant Fischer fetuses therefore developed in a Fischer maternal uterine milieu but the only "maternal" leukocytes to which they were exposed transplacentally were of the alien Lewis type. It was reasoned that if enough of these Lewis cells crossed the placenta and entered the fetus' circulation, they should induce tolerance. To determine whether this had occurred simply required grafting the infants with Lewis skin when they were 21 days old, to see whether their reactivity was impaired. Perfectly healthy litters were born but 50% developed runt or graft-versus-host disease within the first 5 weeks of life and died. Nearly all the survivors gave evidence of unresponsiveness to their Lewis test grafts. Eventually, most of the chimeric mothers also developed the fatal wasting syndrome.

The lymphocytes responsible for initiating runt disease in the baby rats must have been of Lewis origin transmitted from the maternal to the fetal bloodstream across the placenta. Thus, in addition to procuring maternally induced tolerance, we had unwittingly discovered a means of causing maternally induced runt disease. The overt form of this disease was unexpected since, in the usual contexts in which it has been studied (when the putative attacking lymphoid cell inoculum is derived from normal, unsensitized donors), a difference between host and donor at a major histocompatibility locus is mandatory. Lewis and Fischer rats, although differing at four to five histocompatibility loci and capable of rejecting each other's skin grafts within 10 days, are alike at the major (AgB) histocompatibility complex in this species. This suggests that the Lewis lymphoid cell population that the chimeric Fischer mothers transmitted to their fetuses must have acquired an "immune" status. Encouraged by the results of this rather complex experimental procedure, attempts were made to attain similar results by more direct means. Instead of rendering the Fischer females chimeric with the aid of cyclophosphamide before they were mated, we simply took normal Fischer females on the fifteenth day of pregnancy, following mating with males of this strain, and inoculated them intraperitoneally with 200×10^6 lymphoid cells from Lewis rats that had been immunized against Fischer strain tissue antigens. This caused runt disease to develop in 91% of the offspring, though none of the mothers were harmed. Similar results were obtained with other donor-host rat strain combinations, in which the transferred putative "attacking" population of lymphocytes was genetically incompatible both with the fetuses and with the pregnant maternal hosts and against which the latter might reasonably have been expected to react immunologically. At this stage the question arose whether this "foreignness" on the part of the attacking cells with regard to their maternal host was in some way an essential prerequisite for their ability to traverse the placenta in sufficient numbers to harm the fetuses.

To elucidate this important point required yet another modification of the experimental design. For example, we took female Fischer rats and mated them with DA males so that the fetuses were (Fischer × DA)F₁ hybrids, against which the mothers themselves were, at least in theory, capable of reacting immunologically. As we've already seen, however, it is an empirical fact that they do not or cannot exercise this prerogative. On about the fifteenth day of gestation, 200×10^6 lymphocytes were transferred to the mothers from donors of their *own* Fischer strain that had previously been immunized against DA tissue. This again caused a high incidence of runt disease among the progeny.

When females used in this experiment were remated to produce a second litter of hybrid fetuses, the latter usually remained perfectly healthy after birth.

MATERNAL INDUCTION OF RUNT DISEASE FOLLOWING ACTIVE IMMUNIZATION

The high incidence of runt disease among the hybrid progeny of mothers that had been immunized against their fetuses by transfer of living "immune" lymphoid cells from donors of their own strain is difficult to reconcile with the failure of previous attempts to immunize females actively against their hybrid fetuses. To try to resolve this paradox, Fischer females received small skin grafts from DA donors. Then, 1–2 weeks later, when they had rejected these grafts, they were mated with DA males. With this protocol nearly all the progeny succumbed to runt disease. Timing of the active immunization of the mothers was an important factor: grafting 3 weeks before conception was harmless. When actively immunized mothers, whose first litters had succumbed to runt disease, were remated to produce second litters of F_1 hybrids, nearly all of these were born healthy and remained so. Likewise, when normal Fischer females that had given birth to a first litter of (Fischer $\times$ DA)F_1 offspring were immunized with DA skin and subsequently remated with DA males, their progeny were unaffected by runt disease.

A reasonable explanation can be offered for this exemption of second hybrid litters from the disease. As previously mentioned, mothers do eventually make antibodies against some of the important alien histocompatibility antigens of their progeny, though these antibodies are usually not detectable until after a first pregnancy. These antibodies are known to be capable of interfering with both the development and the expression of cell-mediated immunity to allografts or to hosts in graft-versus-host reactions (see Fig. 11-4). That is, these antibodies can fulfill a "blocking" role. Exactly how they do this is still debatable. They may coat the antigenic determinant sites on allogeneic target cells to some extent, thereby concealing them from the attention of "killer" lymphocytes. Also, it has been suggested that, in combination with antigenic material of graft origin, in the form of antigen-antibody complexes, they may also exercise some kind of specific central inhibitory influence on the host's machinery of im-

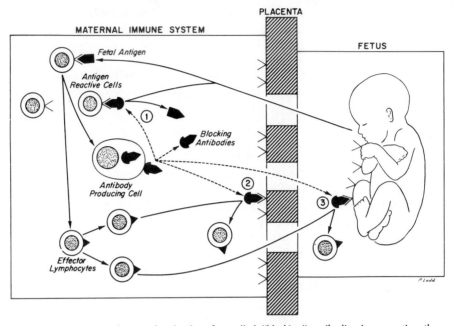

Fig. 11-4. Illustrating the postulated roles of so-called "blocking" antibodies in preventing the development and deployment of a maternal cellular immunity against allogeneic fetal target cells, both in the placenta and within the fetus itself. These antibodies may act (1) by binding to specific antigenic determinants on trophoblastic and other fetal cellular components of the placenta, thus protecting them from destructive engagements with effector or "killer" lymphocytes; (2) by crossing the placenta and binding to antigenic determinant sites on tissues within the fetus, affording it protection against graft-versus-host reactivity on the part of maternal lymphocytes that succeed in crossing the placenta; and, finally, (3) by combining with antigenic material of fetal origin to produce complexes that, by binding at receptor sites on maternal lymphocytes, prevent them from interacting with fetal target cells.

munologic response, producing either a state of tolerance or something closely akin to it that might preclude the production of "killer" or effector lymphocytes by the mothers.

The exemption from runt disease of second litters of hybrid offspring born of mothers which had been actively immunized prior to their first conception and of second litters born of mothers which were not actively immunized until they had already gestated one hybrid litter can reasonably be ascribed to the activity of these "blocking" antibodies. Apart from their possible action within the fetuses at risk, these antibodies may also have acted at the level of the placentas, by combining with, and so masking, the antigenic stimulus that may have played a role in facilitating the passage of lymphocytes from the maternal bloodstream across the placenta.

Is the phenomenon of maternally induced runt disease merely of parochial interest, applicable only to rats, or does it apply in other species as well? Experiments similar in design to those described above have shown that runt disease with high mortality can also be caused in mice, guinea pigs, hamsters, and rabbits by maternal-fetal transmission of lymphocytes across the placenta.

The results of the experiments just described pose some interesting questions. Why have previous investigators been unsuccessful in their attempts to prejudice the survival of fetuses as allografts? In the first place, awareness of the fact that, with the exception of Rh disease in man, untreated females do not normally appear to harm their fetuses immunologically probably prompted them to resort to *hyperimmunization* of the mothers-to-be, by repeated grafting of skin, often with "booster" injections of cell suspensions. This regimen is ideal for stimulating the production of "protective" or blocking antibodies.

Second, if one is looking for an adverse influence of a state of transplantation immunity in a mother directed against her fetuses, one would expect it to occur within the placenta, where tissues of the two individuals are juxtaposed over a very considerable aggregate surface area (about 15 square meters in the 20-week human placenta). Abortions were the results anticipated from such experiments and the consistent birth of apparently healthy litters must have resulted in premature classification of the experiments as unsuccessful. Indeed, it was probably interpreted as supplementary evidence of the completeness of Nature's solution of the allograft problem. Observation of the progeny for a few weeks postpartum might have uncovered the unexpected phenomenon of maternally induced runting.

THE OCCURRENCE OF RUNT OR TRANSPLANTATION DISEASE IN MAN

Soon after it was established that normal, adult, peripheral blood contains immunologically competent cells among its small lymphocyte moiety, attention was drawn to the possibility that runt disease might sometimes occur naturally if enough maternal leukocytes gained access to a genetically appropriate fetus. The risk of causing the disease artificially as a consequence of injecting infants with leukocytes, as for example in attempts to induce tolerance, was also appreciated.

Confirmatory evidence that human infants are indeed susceptible to runt disease was subsequently forthcoming from the untoward results of therapeutic attempts to reconstitute immunologic function in infants with thymic dysplasia and other congenital immunologic deficiency diseases by means of leukocyte or bone marrow cell allografts. Also, in the early days of intrauterine transfusion of packed erythrocytes in the treatment of fetuses severely affected by Rh sensitization in the third trimester, when no attempt was made to render the blood free of leukocytes before transfusion, at least one unequivocal case of fatal runt disease developed.

Close scrutiny of infants who fail to thrive and also present symptoms resembling those of experimentally procured runt disease in animals has produced a few cases of natural, maternally induced runt disease, some even documented by evidence of lymphocyte chimerism. It is also possible that a significant proportion of the fetuses that die *in utero* of "unknown causes" have also been victims of infiltration by their mothers' lymphocytes. There are two factors operating in favor of fetuses: first, the maternal "blocking" antibodies and, second, the fact that in mammals immunologic competence—i.e., ability to react against many kinds of antigen, including those responsible for transplantation immunity, is something that develops long before birth (see Chapter 12). This maturation of immunocompetence in the normally sterile environment in which fetus develops may reflect a protective mechanism that can normally take care of relatively small numbers of potentially harmful immigrant maternal lymphocytes. Indeed, maternal lymphocytes may be the first pathogens to which a fetus is normally exposed! It is perhaps significant that in most cases of established or suspected maternally induced runting in man there was evidence of a congenital immunodeficiency disease in the infant that would have provided the maternal immunocytes the security of tenure needed for them to mount effective reactions against their hosts.

GRAFT-VERSUS-HOST REACTIONS AND LYMPHOMAS

In 1959 two radiologists, Drs. Henry S. Kaplan of Stanford University and Dr. David W. Smithers of London University, drew attention to the marked similarity between the abnormalities of animals suffering from experimentally induced runt disease and those of patients afflicted by certain lymphomas or malignancies of lymphoid tissue. Subsequently it has been shown that mild or even subclinical graft-versus-host reactivity in both mice and rats increases the incidence of lymphomas. Recently Dr. Robert S. Schwartz and his associates at Tufts University School of Medicine have shown that these tumors may arise through the unmasking of latent oncogenic viruses in host cells by the graft-versus-host reactivity. Thus, one must consider the possibility that at least some contribution is made to the relatively high incidence of lymphomas in children by subclinical runt disease, mediated by transplacentally derived maternal lymphocytes. The finding that lymphomas are more frequent among boys than girls parallels our laboratory finding that maternally induced runting is more likely to affect males than females.

REFERENCES

Beer, A. E. 1969. "Fetal erythrocytes in maternal circulation of 155 Rh-negative women." *Obstet. Gynec.* **34**:143–150.

Beer, A. E., and Billingham, R. E. 1973. "Maternally acquired runt disease." *Science* **179**:240–243.

Benirschke, K., and Driscoll, S. G. 1967. *The pathology of the human placenta.* Springer-Verlag, New York, pp. 1–512.

Billingham, R. E., Palm, J., and Silvers, W. K. 1965. "Transplantation immunity of gestational origin in infant rats." *Science* **147**:514–516.

Billingham, R. E., and Silvers, W. K. 1971. *The immunobiology of tissue transplantation.* Prentice-Hall, Englewood Cliffs, N.J.

Breyere, E. J. 1971. "Studies on the permanence of maternal immunological tolerance." *Transplantation* **5**:1504–1509.

Breyere, E. J., and Speiss, P. J. 1973. "Reduction of pre-existing transplantation immunity by specific pregnancy." *Transplantation* **15**:413–415.

Chown, B. 1954. "Anemia from bleeding of the fetus into the mother's circulation." *Lancet* **i**:1213–1215.

Cohen, F., and Zuelzer, W. W. 1967. "Mechanisms of isoimmunization II. Transplacental passage and postnatal survival of fetal erythrocytes in heterospecific pregnancies." *Blood* **30**:796–804.

Currie, G. A. 1970. "The conceptus as an allograft: immunologic reactivity of the mother." *Proc. Roy. Soc. Med.* **63**:61–64.

Diamondopoulos, G. T., and Hertig, A. T. 1963. "Transmission of leukemia and allied diseases from mother to fetus." *Obstet. Gynec.* **21**:150–154.

Jones, E. C., and Krohn, P. L. 1962. "Effect of maternal environment on strain specific differences in ovaries of newborn mice." *Nature* (London) **195**:1064–1066.

Kadowaki, J. I., Zuelzer, W. W., Brough, A. S., Thompson, R. I., Wooley, P. V., and Gruber, D. 1965. "XX/XY lymphoid chimerism in congenital immunological deficiency syndrome with thymic alymphoplasia." *Lancet* **ii**:1152–1156.

Kaplan, H. S., and Smithers, D. W. 1959. "Auto-immunity in man and homologous disease in mice in relation to the malignant lymphomas." *Lancet* **ii**:1–4.

Kleihauer, E., Braun, H., and Betke, K. 1957. "Demonstrations von Fetalem Haemoglobin in den Erythrocyten eines Blutausserichs." *Klin. Wschr.* **35**:637–638.

174   MATERNAL-FETAL EXCHANGE OF CELLS

Lengerová, A. 1957. "Effect of irradiation during embryogenesis on relationship between maternal organism and offspring from aspect of tissue compatibility." *Folia Biol.* (Praha) 3:333–337.

Masouredis, S. P. 1962. "Reaction of I^{131} anti-Rh (D) with enzyme treated red cells." *Transfusion* 2:363–374.

Mollison, P. L., and Hughes-Jones, N. C. 1967. "Clearance of Rh positive red cells by low concentrations of Rh antibody." *Immunology* 12:63–73.

Najarian, J. S., and Dixon, F. J. 1963. "Induction of tolerance to skin homografts in rabbits by alterations of placental permeability." *Proc. Soc. Exp. Biol. Med.* 112:136–138.

Nevanlinna, H. R., and Vainio, T. 1956. "The influence of mother-child ABO incompatibility on Rh immunization." *Vox. Sang.* 1:26–36.

Palm, J. 1974. "Maternal-fetal histoincompatibility in rats: an escape from adversity." *Can. Res.* 34:2061–2065.

Payne, R., and Rolfs, M. E. 1958. "Feto-maternal leukocyte incompatibility." *J. Clin. Invest.* 37:1756–1763.

Peer, L. A., Walia, I. S., and Pullen, R. 1960. "Observations on partial tolerance to skin homografts in man." *Transpl. Bull.* 26:115–118.

Pollack, W., Gorman, J. G., and Freda, V. J. 1969. "Prevention of Rh hemolytic disease." *Prog. Hemat.* 6:121–147.

Pollack, W., Gorman, J. G., Hager, H. J., Freda, V. J., and Tripoli, D. 1969. "Antibody-mediated immune suppression to the Rh factor: Animal models suggesting mechanism of action." *Transfusion* 8:134–145.

Porter J. B., and Breyere, E. J. 1964. "Studies on the source of antigenic stimulation in the induction of tolerance by parity." *Transplantation* 2:246–250.

Potter, J. F., and Shoeneman, M. 1970. "Metastasis of maternal cancer to the placenta and fetus." *Cancer* 25:380–388.

Queenan, J. T. 1967. *Modern management of the Rh problem.* Hoeber Medical Division, Harper & Row, New York, Evanston, and London.

Race, R. R., and Sanger, R. 1969. *Blood groups in man,* 5th ed. Blackwell, Oxford.

Ramseier, H., and Brent, R. L. 1966. "Induction of tolerance to maternal tissue homografts by irradiation of the placenta." *Ann. N.Y. Acad. Sci.* 129:241–249.

Rochna, E., and Hughes-Jones, N. C. 1965. "The use of purified I^{125}-labeled anti gamma globulin in the determination of the number of D antigen sites on red cells of different phenotypes." *Vox. Sang.* 10:675–686.

Rowley, D. A., and Fitch, F. W. 1964. "Homeostasis of antibody formation in the adult rat." *J. Exp. Med.* **120**:987–1005.

Ryder, R. J. W., and Schwartz, R. S. 1969. "Immunosuppression by antibody: Localization of site of action." *J. Immunol.* **103**:970–978.

Salvaggio, A. T., Nigogosyan, G., and Mack, H. C. 1960. "Detection of trophoblast in cord blood and fetal circulation." *Am. J. Obstet. Gynec.* **80**: 1013–1021.

Sanford, B. H. 1963. "Genetic study of modified susceptibility to tumor transplants in reciprocal resistant backcross mice." *J. Nat. Can. Inst.* **31**:169–178.

Schröder, J., Tülikainen, A., and De La Chapelle, A. 1974. "Fetal leukocytes in the maternal circulation after delivery." *Transplantation* **17**:346–354.

Schwartz, R. S. 1972. "Immunoregulation, oncogenic viruses, and malignant lymphomas." *Lancet* **i**:1266–1269.

Stastny, P. 1965. "Accelerated graft rejection in the offspring of immunized mothers." *J. Immunol.* **95**:929–936.

Sterzl, J. 1966. "Immunological tolerance as the result of terminal differentiation of immunologically competent cells. *Nature* (London) **209**: 416–417.

Streilein, J. W., and Grebe, S. 1976. "Graft-versus-host reactions: a review." *Adv. Immunol.* **22**:119.

Sullivan, J. F., and Jennings, E. R. 1966. "Transplacental fetal-maternal hemorrhage." *Am. J. Clin. Path.* **46**:36–42.

Terasaki, P. I., Mickey, M. R., Yamazaki, J. N., and Vredevoe, D. 1970. "Maternal-fetal incompatibility. I. Incidence of HL-A antibodies and possible association with congenital anomalies." *Transplantation* **9**: 538–543.

Tuffrey, M., Bishun, N. P., and Barnes, R. D. 1969. "Porosity of the mouse placenta to maternal cells." *Nature,* London, **221**:1029–1030.

Uhr, J. W., and Baumann, J. B. 1961. "Antibody formation. I. Suppression of antibody formation by passively administered antibody." *J. Exp. Med.* **113**:935–970.

Walknowska, J., Conte, F. A., and Grumbach, M. 1969. "Practical and theoretical implications of fetal/maternal lymphocyte transfer." *Lancet* **i**: 1119–1122.

Woodrow, J. C. 1970. *Rh immunization and its prevention.* Series Haematologica III, 1, Williams & Wilkins, Baltimore.

Woodrow, J. C., and Donohoe, W. T. A. 1968. "Rh-isoimmunization by pregnancy: results of a survey and their relevance to prophylactic therapy." *Brit. Med. J.* **4**:139–144.

Zipursky, A., Pollack, J., Neelands, P., Chown, B., and Israels, L. G. 1963. "The transplacental passage of foetal red blood cells and the pathogenesis of Rh isoimmunization during pregnancy." *Lancet* **ii**:489–493.

Chapter 12

The Ontogeny of the Capacity
to Respond Specifically to Foreign Material

So efficient are the placenta and fetal membranes in protecting, or isolating, the mammalian fetus that only rarely is it unfortunate enough to become inoculated from the maternal circulation or other routes with microorganisms or other antigenic stimuli to which the mother is continuously being exposed. Thus the developing fetus and the newborn animal are normally virtually virgins in an immunologic sense, never having been called upon to respond to an extraneous antigenic stimulus. Birth is followed by immediate contact with large numbers of antigenic determinants as a consequence of establishing respiration, the colonization by intestinal flora, and the absorption of antigenic material associated with food. Exposure to these multiple complex antigens causes a maturation of lymphoid tissue, the "spontaneous" appearance of antibodies of certain types and an increase in the number of cells able to react to certain antigens—i.e., the development of processes that do not occur in the absence of antigenic stimuli.

Despite the existence of long-standing evidence to the contrary, the familiar high susceptibility of infant mammals to infections gave rise to the mistaken and widely held belief that they are highly immature in an immunologic sense—i.e., more or less incapable of responding immunologically against pathogens of a variety of types. Only within the last decade has it become recognized that this susceptibility on the part of the perinate is not due to its immunologic incompetence but rather to a lack of prior "immunologic experience"—i.e., exposure to antigens.

It is now well established that exposure of the newborn to microorganisms does indeed set in motion immune responses of various types, but these are *primary* responses that build up to protective levels slowly. Hence, all too frequently, the pathogens enjoy a sufficient period of virtually unchecked dissemination and proliferation to overwhelm their host. An adult animal who, after being delivered and raised in a germ-free environment, is suddenly thrust into a normal "infected" environment may suffer a similar fate. Of course, the maternal quota of antibodies which the infant normally receives either before or after birth, or both, depending on the species, provides it with a ready-made, highly efficient protective immunologic blanket under the cover of which it gradually acquires its own early immunologic education in the form of primary responses and their legacy of "memory" cells to an ever-increasing number of antigens.

As Drs. Sterzl and Silverstein have pointed out, in a classic review of developmental aspects of immunity, the increasing interest in the maturation of immunologic capability of young animals over the past 20 years has been motivated by two considerations: first, the hope of obtaining evidence supportive of selective theories of the immunologic response and of the *modus operandi* of the phenomenon of immunological tolerance; and, second, recognition that the immunologic status of fetal hosts subject to intrauterine infection may be an important factor affecting the pathogenicity and virulence of the agent and the development of certain congenital malformations.

Experimental Approaches and Sources of Information

As far as experimental animals are concerned, it is obvious that accessibility of the fetus for inoculation, the feasibility of surgical procedures that do not cause interruption of pregnancy, and a reasonably long gestation period are important considerations. One must also be able to recognize whether a given immunity manifested by a fetus following exposure to an antigenic stimulus does indeed reflect an immunologic response on the part of the fetus rather than one manifested by the mother as a consequence of "leakage" of the antigen into her and the subsequent natural passive immunization of the fetuses by antibody transfer antepartum. For this reason a considerable amount of work has been performed on fetal ungulates, particularly sheep, and to a lesser extent cattle, whose placental structure is such as to preclude these possible complications.

In some animals, such as guinea pigs, fetuses can be inoculated directly with antigenic material through the maternal abdomen and uterus prior to birth, enabling an assessment of the recipient's immune status on the day of birth. In fetal lambs, rhesus monkeys, and other species the fetuses can be injected during the latter half of gestation, or even earlier by various routes, including the intravenous and intraperitoneal, and subsequent blood samples or biopsy specimens obtained surgically with low incidence of mortality. A more informative approach involves the introduction of permanent, indwelling catheters into fetal lambs through which antigens can be administered and blood samples withdrawn at regularly spaced intervals, facilitating study of immune elimination of antigen from the fetal circulation and precise determination of the time of appearance of antibodies.

In man, removal of appropriate tissue or cells and cultivation in the presence of antigen or other agents, such as phytohemagglutinin *in vitro,* to test the capacity of the cells to respond affords an important means of evaluating various parameters of lymphoid cell maturation.

Dr. David Rowlands and associates from the University of Pennsylvania are using lethally irradiated (850 r) adult mice reconstituted with defined cell populations prepared from the livers of syngeneic fetal donors of various ages to study the ontogeny of the immune response in this species.

Ontogeny of the Lymphomyeloid Complex in Mammals

Histologic and other studies have shown that the thymus is the first lymphoid organ to develop. In the fetal mouse it is both recognizable and dissectable as an epithelial-mesenchymal rudiment at about 12 days postconception. In the fetal sheep, this stage is reached at about 30–35 days of gestation and thymocytes appear at about 45 days. In man it is an active lymphoid organ at 45 days postconception. The stem cells that proliferate and differentiate in the early thymus are now believed to be of *migratory* origin, coming via the circulation from the yolk sac. As development proceeds, however, an increasing proportion of the lymphoid cells present in the thymus are of bone marrow origin. Within this organ they mature, acquire certain distinctive surface antigens, such as the theta in the mouse, and are subject to continuous release into the circulation as T cells.

Although the precursors of B cells also seem to originate in the embryonic yolk sac, their maturation seems to take place in the liver and bone marrow of the embryo. Development of the latter tissue is still not properly understood. It does seem reasonably certain, however, that bone marrow stem cells are (1) capable of giving rise to B cells, as well as (2) entering the thymus where, as a consequence of division and maturation, they become functional T cells of various types.

In the absence of exposure to antigenic stimuli, the lymphoid tissues of the developing mammalian fetus mature at a very slow rate. The lymphoid tissues of newborn mammals are only moderately cellular, follicular activity is usually absent, and the border between cortex and medulla is indistinct. After birth, however, when the newborn is assailed by a variety of antigenic stimuli, there is a rapid development of the lymphoid tissue system and antibody-synthesizing plasma cells appear. It is interesting to note that in germ-free animals maturation of the lymphoid organs fails to take place. Even in fetal life, precocious maturation of the lymphoid tissues is stimulated by chance natural infection with certain pathogenic microorganisms including those responsible for rubella, toxoplasmosis, and syphilis or by deliberate exposure to a variety of antigenic stimuli, including orthotopic skin allografts.

Clearly antigenic stimulation is responsible for the final stages of maturation of the lymphomyeloid complex of the neonate. In unstimulated fetuses the development of discrete cortical and medullary regions and the appearance of germinal center activity only occur later in gestation. Prior to birth it is restricted to the lamina propria of the intestinal tract and the nodes draining this organ. Presumably this reflects the influence of antigenic stimuli originating within the intestinal lumen. The extensive pioneer work of Silverstein and his associates at Johns Hopkins University Medical School on the fetal lamb *in utero,* together with more limited studies on the young of other species have provided us with a good overall functional picture of the process of immunologic differentiation. Perhaps the most striking and unexpected observation is that competence to react against all antigens is not an attribute that is suddenly acquired by the developing animal. On the contrary, at a particular stage of ontogeny, development of immunological competence proceeds in a *stepwise* manner (see Fig. 12-1). In fetal lambs, of the panel of antigens so far tested, competence to react against the bacteriophage ϕX 174 develops at about 40 days; then, in turn, competence to react against ferritin, skin allografts, and ovalbumin develops sequentially. This developmental sequence does

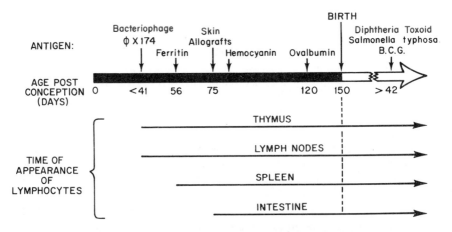

Fig. 12-1. The ontogeny of the capacity to respond to certain defined antigens and the time of appearance of lymphocytes in the various lymphoid tissues of fetal sheep.

not terminate at birth but continues on into the neonatal period. For example, the young lamb does not acquire the ability to react against diphtheria toxoid or *Salmonella* until several weeks after birth.

Silverstein and his associates have shown that for fetal lambs this "hierarchical sequence of immunologic maturation" is remarkably constant from one animal to another, with little temporal variation in the acquisition of the capacity to react against a particular antigen. As far as it goes, the available evidence indicates that equivalent maturation sequences occur in other species including cattle and mice, though of course there are species differences in both the timing and the actual sequence in which competence to react against specific antigens develops.

It is particularly important to note that the fetal lamb at 35–40 days of gestation can form circulating (IgM) antibodies before it has formally organized lymphoid tissues or even many lymphocytes in its body.

Studies on the fetuses of sheep and rhesus monkeys have established that once they have acquired the ability to respond against a given antigen, despite their lymphopenic status, their response presents all the essential components characteristic of the adult response, not only with regard to tempo but also with regard to the classes and heterogeneity of the immunoglobulins produced—IgM and IgG.

In man, *in vitro* studies on fetal tissues have afforded evidence of competence to synthesize IgM and IgG immunoglobulins after the twentieth week of gestation. Various observations indicate that immunoglobulins are normally synthesized before birth even though up to the final month of gestation plasma cells are infrequent in the absence of infection. IgM, which does not cross the placenta, is present in cord blood. The demonstration that, as a consequence of normal pregnancy, some mothers produce antibodies directed against Gm antigens associated with fetal immunoglobulin affords evidence that the normal human fetus is capable of producing IgG molecules having antigenic determinants inherited from the father. These molecules cross the placenta, inducing an immune response in the mother.

Many studies have been conducted upon the antibody responses of newborn human infants because of their relevance to prophylactic immunization procedures. Essentially it appears that normal term, as well as premature, babies can respond by antibody formation to a wide variety of antigens including *Salmonella,* typhoid-paratyphoid, live poliomyelitis vaccine, pertussis, diphtheria, and tetanus; however, there is wide variation in the level of the responses observed. An important contributory factor to this variability is the presence of a high level of maternally acquired antibodies that depress antibody synthesis by the infant to these antigens.

More recent studies of Dr. Hindemann and of Drs. Scott and Beer have highlighted the ability of normal human newborns to respond to erythrocyte antigens of maternal origin. They have demonstrated that some Rh-negative infants born of Rh-positive mothers develop anti-D Rh antibodies shortly after birth (see Chapter 11).

Cellular immunity in man also develops at an early stage of gestation as evidenced by *in vitro* tests making use of transplantation antigens. For example, peripheral blood lymphocytes or spleen cells from 15- to 16-week-old fetuses are stimulated to take up ^{3}H thymidine by exposure to allogeneic lymphocytes or HL-A antigenic material extracted from adult skin. Furthermore, PHA (a potent T cell mitogen) activates lymphoid cells from 16- to 26-week-old fetuses *in vitro*. It is also pertinent to mention that cells that form rosettes with sheep erythrocytes *in vitro*—RFC's, reflecting the presence of immunoglobulin receptors on some lymphocyte surfaces—are present in thymuses from human fetuses of 11 weeks' gestation before such cells appear outside this organ.

In man and other species a factor that has impaired the growth of our knowledge of the ontogeny of delayed hypersensitivity or cellular immune responses in general (excluding the allograft reaction) is the well-documented fact that the skin of the newborn, for partly unknown and nonspecific reasons, affords an unfavorable milieu for inciting delayed inflammatory reactions. That the observed unresponsiveness of its skin to test antigens is not a manifestation of its inability to express a cellular response is indicated by the successful transferability of delayed hypersensitivities from sensitized, newborn pigs and guinea pigs to older normal recipients of their own species.

According to Dr. Richard T. Smith, the factors that may contribute to the diminished capacity of neonatal human skin to develop inflammatory responses include the following: (1) The presence in the challenge site of the neonate of a higher proportion of polymorphonuclear leukocytes and a lower proportion of mononuclear leukocytes during the development of the response compared with the situation in older infants. (2) There is a very high proportion of eosinophils in the infiltrating cell population. (3) The neonate is deficient in IgM opsonins required for efficient phagocytosis. These antibodies begin to appear in the serum 3–6 weeks postpartum. (4) Finally, there is possibly a quantitative deficiency of some of the components of complement.

Obviously the immunological competence of fetal and newborn subjects must depend on many other factors in addition to their ability to summon humoral and cellular immune responses. In man some of the components of complement are synthesized at the beginning of the second trimester of gestation and all the components of complement are demonstrable in 18-week-old fetuses and the process is independent of antigenic stimulation.

In the fetal sheep, the full set of hematologically active components of complement does not appear until the one hundred twenty-fifth day of gestation, there being a rapid increase in level shortly after birth.

THE ONTOGENY OF THE IMMUNE RESPONSE IN MARSUPIALS

Marsupials are born precociously, at a *quasi*-fetal stage of development, and enter the marsupial pouch on the mother's abdomen where they firmly attach themselves to a teat and remain thus for several weeks. For example, young of *Didelphis virginiana,* the Virginia opossum, are born 12.5 days postconception when they weigh about 0.1 g and are equivalent to 9-week human fetuses. At this time they have no circulating lymphocytes and their thymus is no more than a sheet of epithelial cells. Thymic lymphocytes do not appear until the second day of intrapouch life, and lymphocytes appear in the lymph nodes a few days later. The spleen does not acquire its lymphocytes until 17–20 days postpartum. It has been shown that at 5 days postpartum the young can respond to a bacteriophage f2; at 15 days, to a hapten determinant DNP; at 22 days postpartum, to bacteriophage ϕX 174 and *Salmonella typhosa.* Skin allografts transplanted to hosts that were less than 12 days postpartum survived for at least 80 days, but rapid rejection of grafts occurred with older hosts. Thus it appears that in this species, too, the ontogeny of the immune response is a sequential process.

The Australian quokka (*Setonix brachyurus*) has a 28-day gestation period before taking up residence in the maternal pouch. The earliest age at which injections of sheep erythrocytes will elicit an immune response is 10–12 days postpartum.

FETAL IMMUNOCOMPETENCE AND CONGENITAL INFECTIONS

So far we have only considered the ontogeny of immunologic competenence as it applies to harmless antigens used for experimental purposes. We must now consider the type of antigens that naturally confront fetuses as a consequence of congenital infection with complex replicating microorganisms.

Silverstein has recently presented a cogent argument that the transition of the fetus from an immunologically incompetent to an immunologically competent status with regard to a particular pathogenic microorganism may have a profound influence on the host-parasite relationship and the nature of resulting disease processes. For example, an attenuated form of blue tongue virus of sheep is nonpathogenic in adult subjects and is used as a highly effective "live" vaccine which confers protection against subsequent exposure to the wild form of the virus which damages the vascular endothelium. If pregnant ewes are vaccinated, however, their fetuses are infected transplacentally with the attenuated virus and severe damage to their central nervous system results. This fetal susceptibility to the live attenuated virus is restricted to the first half of gestation, during which time it replicates freely and damages susceptible cells. *After* mid-gestation the fetal host seems to be *no more* susceptible to viral damage than an adult sheep, though some multiplication of the virus still occurs. Differentiation of plasma cells occurs at this stage, virus neutralizing antibody appears in the serum, and virus is no longer detectable. The simplest explanation for this changeover from high pathogenicity to absence of pathogenicity of the attenuated virus is the acquisition of competence on the part of the fetus to defend itself immunologically against the viral agent.

By contrast, there are other situations in which, by actually eliciting immune responses, intrinsically innocuous agents cause extensive lesions. A familiar example in adult humans is contact hypersensitivity to poison ivy. The classic fetal model is lymphocytic choriomeningitis virus (LCM) of mice. This virus infects and multiplies within the brains of immunologically incompetent fetal or neonatal hosts doing them no apparent harm; however, infection of immunologically competent normal hosts causes a fatal immunopathologic disease in which the viral antigens constitute the targets of the immunologic attack and host tissues are damaged indirectly as innocent bystanders. The transfer of immunocompetent cells to immunologically incompetent carriers of this virus similarly results in the development of this fatal disease.

Silverstein and Luke's pioneer studies on congenital syphilis in human fetuses indicate that this is probably another example of the same principle. The pathological changes caused by *Treponema pallidum* after it has gained access to the fetus via the placenta are probably not due to any adverse effects that it exerts on host cells but rather to the widespread inflammatory responses and various secondary changes associated with them that it evokes from the host. This inflammatory response may be of an immunologic nature. Infection may occur at an early stage and follow a benign course until the host develops the capacity to respond to the pathogen during the fifth and sixth month of gestation. Silverstein uses the term "modulation" to denote the marked change that occurs in the characteristics of some disease processes as a consequence of maturation of the host's immunocompetence. He cites rubella infection in man as an example. When infection occurs during the first trimester, multiple system congenital anomalies are caused in the absence of any inflammatory response. At this stage the virus seems to exert its effect by interfering with cell division at critical stages of organization rather than by direct pathogenicity. Later in gestation, however, the disease takes the form of chronic inflammatory lesions in which lymphocytes and plasma cells participate. At this stage host reactivity to the viral antigen makes a significant contribution to the pathogenicity. In most instances of congenital rubella the fetuses are damaged by a combination of these two differing disease processes.

Whether immunologic tolerance plays any role in determining the outcome of congenital infection is still open to conjecture. In the late 1930's Traub found that mice exposed *in utero* to LCM virus were unable, in later life, to form neutralizing or complement-fixing antibodies. They became passive carriers of the infection, most of their tissues containing large amounts of infectious virus since every cell type appears to be infected. There is a high level of viremia and virus is excreted in all their secretions. These seemingly unaffected, lifelong passive carriers of the virus transmit it vertically to their own offspring *in utero* and, as congenital carriers, they also show no signs of illness. Thus, at least in the familiar sense of the word, they are "tolerant" of this pathogen. Burnet and Fenner were influenced by this model system when they predicted the phenomenon of immunological tolerance in 1949.

Subsequently, more discriminating studies have yielded evidence that is difficult to reconcile with the thesis that these animals are indeed tolerant of their viral pathogens in an immunologic sense. It has been shown that persistent LCM virus carriers do form antiviral antibody but it is not detectable since it is complexed with viral antigen. Deposition of these antigen-antibody complexes in the kidney leads to disease of the glomeruli. Although the possibility remains that the apparently healthy carrier animals may be tolerant at the level of their cellular immune system, this has yet to be proved. At the moment it appears as though the expression of the cellular immune state is chronically inhibited at the peripheral level by the abundant antigen and/or antigen-antibody complexes; i.e., the phenomenon may indeed be closely similar to that of immunologic enhancement of allografts (see page 124).

Most immunologists now believe that the main contributory factor to absence of unequivocal examples of tolerance of pathogenic microorganisms associated with congenital disease is the antigenic complexity of the organism. Tolerance may exist to some of their components but not to others—a situation that is difficult to document.

A Unifying Concept of the Ontogeny of the Immune Response

At first sight it is exceedingly hard to relate the existing information on the ontogeny of the immune response in different species to specific parameters of development. In his excellent monograph on fetal and neonatal immunology, Dr. J. B. Solomon of the University of Aberdeen presents a percipient analysis of various concepts of *age equivalence* and shows how one variant of them can be applied to enable a meaningful comparison to be made of the development of all species. He develops the thesis that immunocompetence appears at the same "physiological age" in all mammals and birds and reaches the simplifying conclusion that, as far as currently available data go, the onset of the ability to react against transplantation antigens and to synthesize humoral antibodies occur at remarkably similar times on a physiological time scale.

Immunological Competence of the Placenta

In 1962, and subsequently, Dr. Joseph Dancis and various colleagues at New York University Medical Center have published some interesting reports indicative of potential immunological competence and hematopoietic function on the part of the mouse placenta. Initially they claimed that suspensions of cells carefully prepared from the placentas of near-term C57BL/6 fetuses and inoculated into neonatal hosts of the BALB/c strain were almost as effective as spleen cells from adult C57BL/6 donors in causing runt or graft-versus-host disease. Appropriate controls appeared to rule out the possibility that the deaths of the infant mice were caused by infection, the release of toxic factors from placental cells, or (perhaps more plausibly) the presence of contaminating immunocompetent cells of maternal origin. In later publications it was reported that suspensions of placental cells injected into (1) irradiated allogeneic adult mice caused an increased mortality, again suggestive of graft-versus-host reactivity; (2) syngeneic thymectomized newborn mice enhanced their ability to synthesize antibodies against rat erythrocytes; and (3) lethally irradiated syngeneic hosts regularly "seeded" into the spleen, producing nodules comprising both erythroid and lymphoid cellular elements in approximately equal proportions. With the aid of cytologically marked cells it was shown unequivocally that these nodules developed from stem cells present in the cell inocula, though the identity of these cells in the placenta was not established. Some indirect evidence bearing upon this was obtained by carefully fetectomizing mice at 11 days postconception and then removing the placentas to prepare cell suspensions 7 days later when they were almost entirely made up of trophoblast cells. While conceding that small numbers of adventitious cells of varied types and from extraplacental sources in the fetuses may have secreted themselves in the trophoblast as early as the eleventh day of gestation, these workers favored the view that the effects observed were due to the pluripotentiality of trophoblast cells. Unfortunately, critical experiments by other workers, including ourselves, have as yet failed to provide any corroborative evidence of immunocompetence associated with the mouse placenta.

It is pertinent to mention here that although it is commonly believed that mice and rats do not acquire competence to react against antigens (including transplantation antigens) before birth, this is almost certainly not the case. Inoculation of relatively small numbers of allogeneic cells into neonatal hosts may elicit a weak, transient state of sensitivity. The observation that it is almost impossible to induce tolerance of A-strain tissue antigens in C57BL/6 mice by neonatal intravenous injection of relatively high doses of A-strain cells strongly suggests that ability to respond to these antigens must have developed *before* birth or indeed other perinatal influences may be operational in this context (see Chapter 14).

Teleologically, the possession of precocious immunological function within the placenta might confer an important survival advantage upon fetal mammals, protecting them not only against the hazards of microbial infection from their mothers but also against the risk of surreptitious infiltration by maternal leukocytes that, in some genetic contexts, might cause runt disease. Indeed, the first pathogens to which very young mammals are first exposed may be maternal lymphocytes. If there is, in fact, a functional immunologic surveillance system associated with the placenta, it might explain the great rarity with which maternal tumors are transmitted to fetuses in both mice and men. As Benirschke and Driscoll aptly summed up the situation in 1967, "the real role of the placenta as a reactant in infectious diseases and immunity and other defense mechanisms is just beginning to unfold."

REFERENCES

Adinolfi, M. 1972. "Ontogeny of components of complement and lysozyme. In *Ontogeny of acquired immunity*. A Ciba Foundation Symposium. Elsevier, Excerpta Medica, North-Holland, pp. 65–85.

Adinolfi, M., Lessof, M. H. 1972. "Development of humoral and cellular immunity in man." *J. Med. Genet.* 9:86–91.

Auerbach R. 1974. "Development of immunity. In *Concepts of development* (J. Lash and J. R. Whittaker, ed.). Sinauer Associates, Stamford, Conn., pp. 261–271.

Burnet, F. M., and Fenner, F. 1949. *The production of antibodies*. Macmillan, Melbourne.

Dancis, J., Douglas, G. W., and Fierer, J. 1966. "Immunologic competence of mouse placental cells in irradiated hosts." *Am. J. Obstet. Gynecol.* 94:50–56.

188   THE CAPACITY TO RESPOND TO FOREIGN MATERIAL

Dancis, J., Jansen, V., Gorstein, F., and Douglas G. 1968. "Hematopoietic cells in mouse placenta." *Am. J. Obstet. Gynecol.* **100**:1110–1121.

Dancis, J., Samuels, B. D., and Douglas, G. W. 1962. "Immunological competence of placenta." *Science* **136**:382–383.

LaPlanta, E. S., Burrell, R., Watne, A. L., Taylor, D. L., and Zimmermann, B. 1969. "Skin allograft studies in the pouch young of the opossum." *Transplantation* **7**:67–72.

Owen, J. J. T. 1972. "The origins and development of lymphocyte populations." In *Ontogeny of acquired immunity.* A Ciba Foundation Symposium. Elsevier, Excerpta Medica, North-Holland, pp. 35–54.

Rowlands, D. T., Dudley, M. A. 1969. "The development of serum proteins and humoral immunity in opossum 'embryos.' " *Immunology* **17**:969–975.

Schultze, R. D. 1973. "Developmental aspects of the fetal bovine immune response: A review." *Cornell Veterinarian* **63**:507–535.

Silverstein, A. M. 1972. "Immunological maturation in the foetus: Modulation of the pathogenesis of congenital infectious disease." In *Ontogeny of acquired immunity.* A Ciba Foundation Symposium. Elsevier, Excerpta Medica, North-Holland, pp. 17–25.

Silverstein, A. M. 1972. "Fetal immune responses in congenital infection." *N. Eng. J. Med.* **286**:1413–1414.

Silverstein, A. M., and Prendergast, R. A. 1970. "Lymphogenesis, immunogenesis and the generation of immunologic diversity. In *Developmental aspects of antibody formation and structure,* Vol. I (J. Sterzl and I. Riha, ed.). Academic Press, New York, pp. 69–77.

Silverstein, A. M., Prendergast, R. A., and Parshall, C. J. 1970. "Cellular kinetics of the antibody response by the fetal rhesus monkey." *J. Immunol.* **104**:269–271.

Smith, R. T. 1968. "Development of fetal and neonatal immunological function." In *Biology of gestation,* Vol. II (N. S. Assili, ed.). Academic Press, New York, pp. 321–354.

Solomon, J. B. 1971. *Foetal and neonatal immunology.* North-Holland Research Monographs, Vol. 20. Frontiers of Biology. North-Holland, Amsterdam and London.

Sterzl, J., and Silverstein, A. M. 1967. "Developmental aspects of immunity." *Adv. Immunol.* **6**:337–459.

Stites, D. P., Wybran, J., Carr, M. C., and Fudenberg, H. H. 1972. "Development of cellular immunocompetence in man." In *Ontogeny of acquired immunity*. A Ciba Foundation Symposium. Elsevier, Excerpta Medica, North-Holland, pp. 113–129.

Traub, E. 1939. "Epidemiology of lymphocytic choriomeningitis in a mouse stock observed for four years." *J. Exp. Med.* **69**:801–817.

Weiss, L. 1972. *The cells and tissues of the immune system*. Foundations of Immunology Series. Prentice-Hall, Englewood Cliffs, N.J.

Chapter 13

Transmission of Antibodies
from Mother to Offspring Before Birth

Although it has been shown that fetuses can respond immunologically to certain antigens during their sequestered life *in utero* (see Chapter 12), their antigenic experience is normally confined to cells and materials of maternal origin. In respect of these they may become sensitized or immunologically tolerant. Birth, therefore, represents the abrupt confrontation of an infant, who is totally devoid of useful, prior, firsthand immunologic experience, by potentially harmful pathogenic organisms contaminating the environment in which it must spend the rest of its life. Were it not for the fact that the very young mammal receives, by one route or another, "ready-made," the benefit of part of its mother's accumulated repertoire of immunologic experience in the form of passively transferred antibodies, it would almost certainly succumb to massive infection before it could derive any significant protection from actively responding to the microbial antigens concerned. As we shall see in Chapter 14, the vulnerability of colostrum-deprived calves illustrates this situation very dramatically.

This all-important natural, prophylactic, passive immunization of the young may occur (1) before birth; (2) after birth; or (3) during both of these epochs, depending on the species concerned. In primates, rabbits, and guinea pigs, the infants acquire their maternal immunologic endowment before birth by virtue of the ready transmissibility of immunoglobulins of the IgG class across the fetal membranes. At birth the concentration of these antibodies in the infant's circulation is usually similar to, or may even exceed, their concentration in the maternal bloodstream. Expansion of the infant's blood volume, as it grows, in conjunction with the catabolism of the passively transferred antibody molecules, produces a progressive fall in antibody concentration. The eventual rise in antibody level reflects the coming into operation of the subject's own immunologic defense machinery. Little if any *systemic* passive immunization occurs after birth in these species since the gut is incapable of transmitting antibodies from colostrum or milk.

190

In mice, rats, cats, and dogs this all-important process of natural passive immunization with maternal antibody takes place *after* birth, as well as before this event, the greater contribution coming from the breast via its exosecretion. In ungulates, by contrast, transmission only occurs immediately after birth.

The subject matter of this chapter is a consideration of the transmission of antibody *before* birth. Transmission of antibody after parturition will be dealt with in Chapter 14.

Transmission of Antibodies in the Rabbit

With regard to the transmission of immunity from mother to fetus we have more information on the rabbit than on other species on account of its availability and suitability for experiments involving surgical procedures on the pregnant uterus. Since both humans and rabbits have placentas of the hemochorial type, in which the maternal uterine endometrium is eroded so that the trophoblast-covered fetal villi are bathed in lakes of maternal blood, it was for long tacitly assumed that in both species immunity was transmitted by the same route—i.e., across the placenta.

The work of the late Professor F. W. Rogers Brambell of University College, Bangor, Wales, and his "school," and also of other investigators, has established that both homologous and heterologous plasma proteins—including actively and passively acquired antibodies—pass fairly readily and on a nondiscriminatory basis from the circulation of a pregnant rabbit through the bilaminar omphalopleur, which forms the wall of the large yolk sac, into the yolk sac fluid on the seventh, eighth, and probably ninth day after copulation. At this time the fetal heart begins to beat and the vitelline circulation to the yolk sac is established.

Transmission of maternal antibody to the fetus continues after the disruption of the bilaminar wall of the yolk sac, which occurs on about the sixteenth day after copulation. This is evidenced, first, by a continuous rise in the fetal serum content of circulating maternal bacterioagglutinins and hemagglutinins from the twenty-second day of gestation to term and, second, by the finding that if pregnant rabbits are actively immunized to *Brucella abortus* after the fifteenth day of gestation, the young at birth have titers of serum antibodies closely resembling those of the maternal sera.

The route by which this maternal antibody is transmitted was established by an elegant experimental study by Brambell and his associates. Two possibilities merited their serious consideration: (1) Transmission of immunity occurs directly across the placenta, as most people believed, or (2) it occurs as a consequence of direct antibody secretion from the maternal circulation into the uterine lumen, its subsequent uptake by the inverted yolk sac splanchnopleur and eventual transportation to the fetus by the vitelline circulation supplying the yolk sac.

First, these investigators demonstrated that antiserum to *Brucella* inoculated into the lumen of one uterine horn of a pregnant rabbit on the twenty-fourth day of gestation was present, 24 hours later, in the sera of all fetuses from the inoculated horn but *not* in the sera of those from the uninoculated horn. Second, they found that by placing sutures around the yolk sac stalk, without perforating the membrane, the circulation through the area vasculosa of the yolk sac splanochnopleur could be interrupted. When this was done, it prevented the uptake by the experimentally treated fetuses of antibodies injected into the lumen of the ipsilateral uterine horn or into the mother's bloodstream. It was also established that antibodies are present in the uterine fluid of nonpregnant animals though at a lower concentration than in the maternal serum. Taken together, these experiments afford conclusive proof that, in the rabbit, passive immunity is not acquired by the fetuses via the placenta but by absorption from the uterine lumen into the embryonic circulation of the area vasculosa of the yolk sac wall.

SELECTIVITY OF MATERNAL-FETAL TRANSMISSION OF ANTIBODIES IN RABBITS

Before discussing the selectivity of the antibody transmission process a brief outline of the principal immunoglobulins will be helpful. This relates to the immunoglobulin system of man because at present this is better defined and understood than that of any other species.

IgG is the dominant serum immunoglobulin. It has a molecular weight of 160,000 and a sedimentation constant of 7S; it is comprised of four polypeptide chains, two light and two heavy. Unlike immunoglobulins of the other classes it can cross the placenta in some species.

IgM is the largest of the immunoglobulin molecules, having a molecular weight of 900,000 and a sedimentation constant of 19S. It, too, has the basic 4-chain structure—two light and two heavy chains, but groups of 5 of these are united together to form a 20-chain (i.e., a 5 × 4) molecule. These antibody molecules are highly efficient in agglutinating red cells and bacteria.

IgE, the most recently discovered class of immunoglobulin molecules, is present in small amounts in serum. It has a molecular weight of 196,000, binds to surface receptors on mast cells and basophilic leukocytes, and is responsible for immediate hypersensitivity and allergic reactions.

IgA immunoglobulin molecules as found in the serum are primarily 7S with a molecular weight of 170,000 and comprised of 4 polypeptide chains. About 10% of the molecule is composed of carbohydrate. What has been designated as *secretory* IgA antibody is found in almost all external secretions of the body where it constitutes the dominant immunoglobulin. Secretory IgA has a molecular weight of 390,000 and a sedimentation coefficient of 11S. It consists of dimers of serum IgA plus an additional nonimmunoglobulin component having a molecular weight of 50,000–60,000 called secretory "piece." This latter seems to be produced in epithelial cells rather than in the immunoglobulin-producing plasma cells.

IgA molecules are synthesized by plasma cells located in the mucous membranes, beneath the epithelia. They may then enter the general circulation and form part of the serum IgA pool, or they may pass across the membranes of nearby epithelial cells where they acquire the *locally* synthesized secretory piece (sometimes referred to as *transport* piece). The complete secretory IgA molecules are then secreted from the apical ends of the epithelial cells. It has recently been shown that the mucosal epithelial cells of the gastrointestinal tract actually store secretory IgA that is released as they slough.

Irrespective of their class, e.g., whether IgG or IgM, all antibodies produced by female rabbits seem to be transmitted with equal facility to the circulation of their fetuses, either following inoculation into the uterine cavity or injection into the maternal circulation. By contrast, rabbit albumin is less readily transmitted and the serum α and β globulins are only transmitted in small amounts. However, the yolk sac displays marked selective transmission of both antibodies and other serum proteins from *alien* donor species. For example, the transmission of rabbit antitoxins is about 100 times greater than that of bovine antitoxins and the transmission of human antitoxins is superior to those of guinea pigs.

With the aid of "labeled" Fc and Fab fragments of papain-digested rabbit IgG it has shown that the Fc piece is transmitted from the uterine cavity to the fetal circulation almost as readily as the intact antibody molecule, whereas transmission of the Fab piece occurs at a much lower rate. These findings suggests that the Fc piece of rabbit γ globulin, which lacks antibody activity but retains much of the antigenicity of the intact molecule, is primarily responsible for the transmission, probably by acting as a "recognition" unit that determines the acceptability of the molecule for uptake and transmission by cells of the fetal yolk sac.

TRANSMISSION OF IMMUNITY IN MICE AND RATS

In mice and rats, although some immunity is transmitted before birth, most of the transmission takes place via the colostrum and milk postpartum. Before birth a variety of antibodies are transmitted, probably even earlier than the eighteenth day of gestation. In the rat it has been shown that the yolk sac and vitelline circulation is an important route of transmission though some transmission seems to occur across the placenta.

In the guinea pig, which also has a hemochorial type of placenta, a wide variety of antibodies are transmitted before birth and the level of antitoxins in the serum of the newborn young is usually at least twice that in the maternal serum. Here, too, it has been shown that the transmission route is by way of the yolk sac and vitelline circulation.

MATERNAL → FETAL TRANSFER OF ANTIBODIES IN PRIMATES

Two completely independent areas of investigation in man have resulted in an extensive literature documenting the transmission of immunity: (1) comparison of the antibody concentration (usually to toxins, actively or passively acquired by the mother) in the cord blood of newborn infants with that of their mothers and (2) studies on hemolytic disease of the newborn (see Chapter 11).

In the primates in general both the development and the final structures of the placenta and fetal membranes differ markedly from those of the species we've considered so far and of course considerable interspecific differences exist. The allantoic cavity is vestigial, the yolk sac is mere rudiment, and there are other important anatomical differences too involved to be considered here. The discoid placenta is hemochorial but of the lacunar type, being very different from the hemochorial placenta of the rabbit. On purely anatomical grounds, transmission of immunity could not take place via the vascular splanchnic wall of the yolk sac as it does in rabbits, guinea pigs, and rats.

Since the chorion forms a complete boundary between maternal and fetal tissue at all points, transmission must occur across it and the question is whether the antibodies traverse the chorionic trophoblast within the placenta or whether they cross the chorion laeve. The most obvious and direct route is from the maternal bloodstream in the placental lacunae, across the layer of trophoblast covering the villi to the abundant fetal capillaries within them. Although, as we shall see, the route of transfer is predominantly by the latter route, Brambell and his associates were initially very much attracted by the possibility that some transfer might take place via the amniotic fluid. The fetuses swallow this on a more or less continuous basis and various substances, including antibodies, could be absorbed from it by the fetal gut and so enter the circulation. The appeal of this particular route for the transmission of immunity, of course, is that it would involve absorption by endoderm, which seems to occur in all other groups of animals. Antibodies, as well as other substances, could gain access to the amniotic fluid either from the maternal blood in the placental lacunae across the chorionic plate of the placenta and its covering of amnion or from blood in the vessels of the decidual lateralis, the remnants of the uterine lumen, and the chorion laeve with its lining of amnion.

There is a copious literature documenting the transmission of a wide variety of antibodies to a wide range of antigens of a bacterial and viral nature as well as to platelets and leukocytes, from actively immunized mothers. Information on the transmission of immunity passively acquired by the mother is still very sparse, however. Despite the range of antibodies that are transmitted antepartum, the process of transmission is highly selective with regard to the class of immunoglobulin that is transmitted. IgG molecules are readily transmitted, whereas those of IgM and IgA are not. That IgE is not transferred is evidenced by the failure of transfer of reaginic antibodies in spite of high titers in the maternal serum.

The failure of IgM to transfer may be related to its high molecular weight of 900,000, but the failure of IgA to transfer cannot be ascribed simply to its molecular weight since the monomeric form of this immunoglobulin has a molecular weight that is closely similar to that of IgG.

The presence in the amniotic fluid of immunoglobulin of maternal origin (and other proteins too) has long been recognized and its significance has been a subject of conjecture. The observations that ABO blood group substances (in the case of secretor mothers) and Gc proteins were present in amniotic fluid but not in fetal serum suggested that they must have come from the maternal circulation by the direct route—i.e., by transmission across the chorion.

As far as the monkey is concerned, the most telling evidence in favor of the placenta being the principal route of transmission was obtained by Dr. D. R. Bangham and his associates at the National Institute for Medical Research in London. They injected labeled homologous serum proteins intravenously into pregnant monkeys 8–9 hours before Caesarean section. Although albumin and γ globulins were transmitted to the fetal plasma, the γ globulin was transmitted 10–20 times more rapidly than the albumin and only very small amounts of α and β globulin were transmitted. Labeled albumin and a very small amount of globulin were also present in the amniotic fluid. In a subsequent experiment, labeled homologous serum was injected directly into the amniotic cavity of fetal monkeys and sequential samples of maternal and fetal serum and of amniotic fluid were taken at intervals thereafter. Only evidence of the swallowing of the labeled protein from the amniotic fluid was obtained—it was present in high concentration in the contents of the duodenum and the jejunum— and only very small amounts of the labeled proteins were demonstrable in the fetal serum after 24 hours.

These experiments constitute strong evidence that the placenta is the principal route of transmission in the monkey. Supportive evidence was subsequently presented by Dr. Leslie Quinlivan of the University of Pittsburgh, who injected labeled homologous globulin into monkeys during the last four weeks of gestation and obtained evidence that the amount of γ globulin in the maternal serum rose with time over a 5-day, postinjection observation period. The amount of labeled γ globulin in the amniotic fluid remained more or less constant at a fairly low level.

Experiments have also been performed on human subjects. These have entailed injection of labeled homologous serum albumin or γ globulin intravenously into pregnant women or into the amniotic cavities of their fetuses approximately 24 hours before termination of their pregnancies by Caesarian section. In other experiments, labeled homologous proteins were injected into normal pregnant women during the final month of pregnancy. When pregnancy was terminated, or ended naturally in these experiments, samples of maternal blood, cord (i.e., fetal) blood, and amniotic fluid were taken and assayed for their content of labeled material. The results also indicated direct transmission of the labeled material to the fetal blood via the placenta rather than indirectly via the amniotic cavity.

An additional observation pertaining to the route of transmission of immunity in man comes from a study of newborn infants with esophageal atresia who had therefore been incapable of swallowing amniotic fluid. These infants were found to have diphtheria antitoxin levels that were similar to those in the serum of their mothers.

In the light of all the available evidence it is clear that the principal route of transmission of immunity in primates is via the placenta. Although there is no doubt that serum proteins, including antibodies, do reach the amniotic fluid from which they are transmitted to the fetal bloodstream, this process is slow and of trivial magnitude.

REFERENCES

Note: The references at the end of Chapter 14 should also be consulted.

Bangham, D. R. 1960. "The transmission of homologous serum proteins to the foetus and to the amniotic fluid in the rhesus monkey." *J. Physiol.* **153**:265–289.

Bangham, D. R., Hobbs, K. R., and Terry, R. J. 1958. "Selective placental transfer of serum-proteins in the rhesus." *Lancet* **ii**:351–354.

Barnes, J. M. 1959. "Antitoxin transfer from mother to foetus in the guinea pig." *J. Path. Bact.* **77**:371–380.

Brambell, F. W. R. 1970. *The transmission of passive immunity from mother to young.* American Elsevier Publishing Co., New York.

Cohen, S. 1971. "The structure and biological properties of antibodies." In *Immunological diseases.* (M. Samter, ed.). Little, Brown and Co., Boston, pp. 39–65.

Dancis, J. 1960. "Transfer of proteins across the human placenta." In *The placenta and fetal membranes* (C. A. Villee, ed.). Williams & Wilkins Co., Baltimore, pp. 185–187.

Dancis, J., Lind, J., Oratz, M., Smolens, J., and Vara, P. 1961. "Placental transfer of proteins in human gestation." *Am. J. Obstet. Gynecol.* **82**: 167–171.

Quinlivan L. G. 1967. "Gama globulin-^{131}I transfer between mother and off-spring in the rhesus monkey." *Am. J. Physiol.* **212**:324–328.

Solomon, J. B. 1971. *Foetal and neonatal immunology.* North-Holland Publishing Co., Amsterdam and London.

Tomasi, T. B. 1971. "The gamma A globulins: First line of defense." In *Immunobiology* (R. A. Good and D. W. Fisher, ed.). Sinauer, Stamford, Conn., pp. 76–83.

Wasz-Hockert, O., Wager, T., Hautala, T., and Widholm, O. 1956. "Transmission of antibodies from mother to foetus. A study of the diphtheria level in the newborn with oesophageal astresia." *Ann. Med. Exp. Biol. Fenn.* **34**:444–446.

Chapter 14

Transmission of Antibodies
from Mother to Offspring After Birth:
The Immunological Significance of the Mammary Gland,
with Special Reference to Its Products

Mammary glands are of immunologic significance for a variety of reasons, both clinical and veterinary, some of which are well-known and others of which are only now emerging. For example: (1) Mammary glands secrete antibodies that are taken up and may be concentrated from the serum on a highly selective basis. (2) Antibody formation may actually occur *locally* within the mammary glands in some species. However the ability of the infants of some species, notably man, to derive any benefit from this postpartum passive immunization has only recently been established. (3) In some species ingestion of colostral antibodies from mothers sensitized to fetal isoantigens during pregnancy may have fatal consequences for the newborn. (4) Colostrum and milk include certain unique or distinctive ingredients that are potentially autoantigenic for both the secretor and the recipient and are therefore potential causes of unwanted or even harmful immunologic responses. (5) Both colostrum and milk normally contain significant numbers of *living* leukocytes the presence and significance of which has been almost totally neglected. Apart from their possible action as alloantigens, these cells may confer immunologic benefits upon the recipients or, in certain genetic contexts, might even represent threats to their well-being.

The purpose of this chapter is to review the immunobiology of lactation from both the maternal and the suckling's point of view.

THE ANTIBODY CONTENT OF COLOSTRUM AND MILK
AND ITS ORIGIN

Recognition that the exosecretion of mammary glands contains antibodies, or at least important protective agents, and that these confer striking benefits upon the young of some species, notably cattle, is almost as old as immunology itself. In the absence of a colostral supply newborn calves often succumb very rapidly to an intestinal bacterial disease due to *Escherichia coli* and known as "white scours." Ingestion of very small amounts of colostrum or serum gives protection. In 1892 Paul Ehrlich demonstrated, on the basis of foster nursing experiments in mice, that suckling from mothers immunized with abrin or ricin, two potent phyto-toxins, conferred some measure of resistance to subsequent challenge with these agents. He also established that antibodies passively transferred to lactating mothers are likewise transmissible to their progeny by suckling. Subsequently a tremendous amount of work has been devoted to the anti-body content of colostrum and milk, its secretion, the completeness with which it reflects the mother's prior immunologic experience, and (more recently, with the aid of newer techniques) the extent to which the various classes of immunoglobulin molecules present in her serum are secreted by mammary glands. Finally, and most importantly, there is the question of the usefulness of the product from the infant "consumer's" viewpoint.

In cattle, sheep, goats, and rabbits, antibodies in high concentration appear to be transmitted *unchanged,* i.e., without degradation and re-synthesis, from the maternal plasma to the lacteal secretions, and this con-clusion is consonant with evidence of a decline in serum gamma globulin levels at the time of colostrum formation. In 1961 Dr. Frank Dixon and his associates of the Scripps Clinic and Research Foundation at La Jolla demonstrated the ability of the bovine mammary acinar epithelium to dis-tinguish between gamma globulins and the smaller molecules of albumin, in that it preferentially takes up and transfers into the secretion more of the former than of the latter. These investigators also made the important observation that in cows, at the time of parturition, the average gamma globulin concentration in colostrum is five times that of the serum. When heterologous gamma globulin of human origin is transferred to lactating cows, it too is taken up, concentrated, and secreted by the mammary gland. Histologic, histochemical, and electron microscopic studies revealed few plasma cells in the colostrum-forming udders of apparently healthy cows and gave no convincing evidence of *local* gamma globulin synthesis. It is generally recognized, however, that pathologic processes may lead to accumulation of plasma cells in the udder and so alter this situation.

Subsequent discriminatory biophysical and immunological studies on bovine immunoglobulins have shown that the mammary gland selectively transports certain classes of antibody from the plasma to the colostrum. Like those of other species, bovine immunoglobulins comprise a hetero-geneous population of molecules, divisible into a number of classes and subclasses on the basis of molecular size, structure, and physical and biological properties.

The predominant immunoglobulins in the serum of ruminants are closely similar components, IgG_1 and IgG_2, present in approximately similar concentrations and having almost identical physical and other properties. They differ with regard to their electrophoretic mobilities, the IgG_1 being the faster moving. About 5 weeks before parturition, however, the concentration of IgG_1 in the mammary secretion is about 11 times higher than that of IgG_2. Furthermore, 2–3 weeks before parturition there is an abrupt decrease in the concentration of IgG_1 in the maternal serum; yet during this period the concentrations of the other serum immunoglobulins remain unchanged. The concentrations of IgM and IgA in the colostrum just prior to or immediately after parturition are 5 to 7 times higher than those in the serum, however, indicating the ability of mammary epithelium to concentrate these immunoglobulin molecules also.

Comparative studies of the immunoglobulins present in the various exosecretions of cattle have revealed a striking disparity between the products of "normal" secretory glands such as salivary, lacrimal, and prostate and the nasal and intestinal mucosas on the one hand and the mammary gland on the other hand. In the first series secretory IgA, synthesized locally by the plasma cells, is the major immunoglobulin present. In the mammary gland exosecretion, however, as we've just seen, the predominant immunoglobulin is IgG_1, which is selectively taken up and transported from the serum. Nevertheless secretory IgA is a definite though minor component of both bovine colostrum and milk. Of special interest is the observation that milk contains a relatively large amount of the free secretory "piece," believed to be synthesized by mammary epithelial cells.

In pigs and horses, too, secretory IgA either does not occur in colostrum or makes only a minor contribution to its total immunoglobulin content, IgG being the major constituent. In rats, whereas IgA is only a trace immunoglobulin in the serum, what appears to be its secretory form is the dominant immunoglobulin in the colostrum. In the rabbit the serum contains only about 200 μg ml of IgA, comprising slightly less than 2% of the total circulating immunoglobulins; yet in the colostrum secretory IgA predominates, having a concentration of 3–4.5 mg/ml. An *in vitro* study on mammary tissue from lactating rabbits has shown that the T chains of secretory IgA are synthesized locally and provided suggestive evidence that the IgA molecules to which they are attached are derived from the serum.

As recently as 1970, Brambell drew attention to the fact that relatively little attention had been paid to the immunology of human colostrum and milk as compared with that devoted to the similar bovine secretions. In general it may be stated that in man there are large differences in the extent to which a given serum antibody is secreted into the colostrum and milk. Antibodies with specificities to enteric organisms are preferentially secreted. Small amounts of diphtheria antitoxin—always less than in the maternal serum—are present in the colostrum of actively immunized mothers 48–60 hours postpartum but are not detectable in milk after about 60 hours. Typhoid H and O agglutinins are also demonstrable in colostrum, sometimes in greater concentrations than in the serum; however, both soon disappear from the milk. Milk, too, contains immunoglobulins with antibody activity against several microorganisms including *Escherichia coli,* the most important pathogen of the neonate. It also contains isoagglutinins corresponding to the ABO blood group system, as well as Rh antibodies, sometimes in high titer.

About 15 years ago, the important discovery was made that in man secretory IgA is the predominant immunoglobulin present in milk as well as in other external secretions. The early colostrum may contain as much as 20–40 mg/ml of secretory IgA but this drops to about 1 mg/ml after a few days; however, increase in milk production compensates for this fall in concentration. Small amounts of IgG and IgM are also present in milk. Although not yet proved, it seems very likely, in view of the abundance of plasma cells associated with active mammary glands in man, that the IgA secreted is synthesized *locally* rather than being transferred from the serum.

Mode of Secretion of Antibodies by the Mammary Gland

The ability of the mammary gland to select, concentrate, and transmit to colostrum serum proteins, and especially immunoglobulins, from the heterogeneous maternal serum pool raises the intriguing question of the mechanism(s) involved. Ultrastructural studies have established the intimate apposition of adjacent alveolar epithelial cells near their apical ends by tight junction-like zones, tending to preclude the possibility of transfer via the intercellular spaces. Rather, transfer of IgG and other protein molecules probably occurs *through* the epithelial cells within transport vesicles. Dr. M. R. Brandon and his associates of the Dairy Research Unit at Sydney University in Australia have made the interesting suggestion that in cattle the selective transfer of IgG_1 relative to IgG_2 into the colostrum may turn upon the presence of receptor sites on the basal or intercellular membranes of glandular epithelial cells, so that transport vesicles developing at these sites would contain more IgG_1 than IgG_2.

In cattle, sheep, goats, horses, donkeys, and pigs, maternal antibodies are virtually unable to cross the maternal-fetal barrier *in utero* and the young derive their entire complement of maternal antibodies from the concentrate in colostrum during the first few hours of life. The transmission of these colostral antibodies across the gut to the infant's circulation is an extremely rapid process, frequently being confined to a very short time interval. For example, colostrum or serum antibody fed orally to calves more than 48 hours postpartum fails to benefit them since the antibodies undergo digestion and degradation before absorption.

In rats, mice, cats, and dogs, as mentioned previously, this all-important passive immunization with maternal antibodies takes place after birth as well as before this event, the greater contribution coming from the breast via the colostrum and milk. Unlike the situation in ungulates, in these species intestinal absorption of antibodies from colostrum and milk continues for a significant portion of lactation.

In humans, transfer of antibodies from mother to child occurs almost exclusively across the placenta, and only antibodies of one class, IgG, are transmitted. Although antibodies are present in both colostrum and milk, none of them are absorbed from the infant's gut. For example, in no case have Rh antibodies been detected in the sera of infants fed with milk or serum containing a high titer of these antibodies. Likewise, no significant absorption of ABO isoagglutinins takes places from the gut.

As this seemingly paradoxical state of affairs became well substantiated, in the minds of many, the advocates of breast feeding had lost one of their strongest arguments. For example, in 1956 Vahlquist wrote . . . "available data refute the concept that human milk is of any appreciable importance as a source of protective antibodies for the child." The assumption here, of course, was that if maternal antibodies cannot gain access to the infant's bloodstream and body fluids, they can do it no good. The idea that antibodies might fulfill an important function *locally* within the lumen of the gastrointestinal tract was almost completely neglected. Here the situation stood for a few years until, with the aid of new techniques, the important discovery was made that secretory IgA is the predominant immunoglobulin in milk as in other external secretions of man, including those of parotid gland, saliva, tears, nasal, and tracheobronchial secretions. Since this immunoglobulin is believed to play an antimicrobial protective role for the mucous membranes across whose epithelium it is secreted, it was suggested that, in humans, milk antibodies do indeed fulfill an important protective function partly by acting *locally* within the lacteal ductal system of the mammary gland but principally in the gastrointestinal tract of the infant. There is now a considerable body of circumstantial evidence supporting this premise—for example: (1) Breast milk does contain secretory IgA-type antibodies against *Escherichia coli*. (2) Apart from a wealth of clinical evidence that breast-fed babies are less prone to enteric infections than bottle-fed babies, correlations have been discovered between the levels of antibodies to *Escherichia coli* in human colostrum and the number of coliform bacteria in the stools of breast-fed newborn. (3) Breast feeding interferes with the effectiveness of oral polio-virus vaccination. (4) The secretory IgA molecule is more resistant to pH changes and to proteolytic enzymes than is either serum IgA or other immunoglobulins, which may enable secretory IgA molecules to function in the milieu of the gut. (5) That such antibodies are demonstrable in the stools (copro-antibodies) is direct evidence of their capacity to withstand digestive processes. So far, the manner in which IgA exerts its antimicrobial action has not been discovered. It has been suggested that it may act by preventing the attachment of bacteria to cells on mucosal surfaces and so preventing their penetration into the tissues. It may also neutralize toxins liberated within the lumen of the gut.

The well-established superiority of human milk over that of the cow in protecting the newborn against infection almost certainly turns in part upon its higher content of secretory IgA-type antibodies against pathogenic bacteria peculiar to man.

ADVERSE EFFECTS OF COLOSTRUM AND MILK DUE TO THEIR ANTIBODY CONTENT

Despite their important survival value for mammals, neither colostrum nor milk is entirely beneficent from the viewpoint of the infant recipient.

Members of those species that receive their maternal immunologic endowment exclusively via the colostrum and milk *after* birth are not necessarily exempt from the risk of hemolytic disease of the newborn. Jaundice of newborn foals has long been recognized as a serious and usually rapidly fatal disease among mules. Two French investigators, Drs. Caroli and Bessis, demonstrated in 1947 that this disease is closely similar to *erythroblastosis fetalis* in man. Mares that have given birth to affected mule foals consistently give birth to affected foals following subsequent mating with donkeys. If mated with horses, however, they produce perfectly healthy offspring. Affected mule foals are perfectly healthy at the time of birth and the symptoms of the disease—agglutination of their red cells, frequently hematuria, and jaundice—usually do not develop until a few hours postpartum. Death ensues within a day or two. In all instances the mother's blood, milk, and colostrum contain a high titer of antibodies directed against both donkey and mule erythrocytes, and the red cells of all affected mules give positive antiglobulin reactions that are indicative of their being coated with immunoglobulin. The cause of this disease is, first, immunization of the mare against certain *donkey-specific* red cell antigens that her mule fetus inherited from its father and, second, transfer of these antibodies, via the colostrum, to the infant mule after birth. The severity of the disease is related to the antibody titer of the colostrum. Prevention of the newborn mule foal from receiving colostrum from its mother until after she's been milked for a few days obviates the disease since, although the harmful antibodies are still present in her milk, the offspring's ability to absorb them is of very short duration.

Hemolytic disease of the newborn of similar etiology also occurs in thoroughbred horses and pigs. Here, of course, the red cell antigens involved are *isoantigens,* i.e., those whose determinant genes are segregating within the species concerned.

Although Rh antibodies may be present in high titer in both the colostrum and milk of lactating women, their presence poses no threat to a genetically susceptible neonate because of its inability to absorb them from its gut. Thus there is no risk whatsoever associated with nursing an Rh-positive infant by a sensitized Rh-negative woman.

The Antigenic Status of Milk
and Its Possible Adverse Consequences

By virtue of its variety of complex protein constituents it is scarcely surprising that at least 18 distinct antigenic specificities are recognizable serologically when colostrum from one species is inoculated into a recipient of an unrelated species—e.g., from cow into rabbit. Fewer antigenic determinants (10–11) are associated with milk. These specificities are probably all species-specific—i.e., present in colostrum and milk from *all* members of the donor species but not represented in the milk from the reacting, alien host species.

Colostrum and milk also include *unique* ingredients such as casein, which are synthesized and secreted by mammary glands during lactation and are found nowhere else in the body. Since females do not produce milk until long after their immunologic machinery has attained functional maturation, there is a *prima facie* case that they might be capable of reacting immunologically against some of their *own* milk proteins, and possibly even of damaging the cells that secrete them because of the lack of opportunity to become tolerant of them during early life. That females do not normally become immunized to their own milk may be attributable to the sequestered status of this exosecretion from its synthesis to its ejection: It does not normally enter the draining lymphatic system and gain access to the circulation, so that the host's immunologically competent cells do not become exposed to it.

Experiments conducted upon goats and rabbits have established the isoantigenicity of milk proteins—i.e., the ability of milk from one individual to elicit an immune response in an unrelated recipient to the *same* species. A limited number of findings have also established the potential *autoantigenicity* of milk. In 1934 Lewis showed that goats can make antibodies to their own casein, and more recently Dr. K. Bratanov of the Institute of Biology and Pathology of Reproduction in Sofia, Bulgaria, has reported that if a lactating rabbit is inoculated with as little as 1 ml of its *own* milk and this procedure is repeated about 10 days later, a fatal anaphylactic reaction results. He also found that inoculation of goats and sheep with their *own* milk incited the production of low titers of antibody.

In humans, rare cases of women who developed a serum sickness-like illness following rapid absorption of their own milk have been reported, as well as one of a woman who developed a strong immediate type cutaneous hypersensitivity to her own milk. Dr. Von Amman and his associates in Bern, Switzerland, claim that in about one-fifth of all women rapid cessation of lactation is followed by the appearance of hemagglutinating and complement-fixing antibodies directed against antigens in human milk. Although no one so far has succeeded in producing autoimmune mastitis in any experimental animal, in the light of the evidence cited above it is conceivable that some forms of mastitis in women might have an autoimmune etiology. Finally, it may be emphasized that, at least in theory and perhaps depending very much on their genetic constitution, babies could become allergic to their mother's milk, just as a few unfortunate women have been shown to develop dramatic allergic reactions to their husband's (or other donor's) seminal plasma (see page 68).

Milk Allergy

Among antigens responsible for clinically overt, distressing allergic symptoms after ingestion of food, cow's milk ranks high on the list, particularly in children, among whom allergic manifestations may be as high as 6%. Careful studies with fractionated milk proteins have implicated 4 different antigens—α-lactoalbumin, β-lactoglobulin, casein and bovine serum albumin—about equally as the allergic components responsible. There are good grounds for belief that many of the "rashes" and skin lesions so common in infants are manifestations of local, "immediate" type allergic responses to some of the heterologous protein antigens present in their "formula" diet. If this is true, infants exclusively sustained by their mother's milk should have a lower incidence of these troublesome skin lesions.

Cot or Crib Death

One of the important enigmas of pediatrics is the sudden infant (or crib) death syndrome (SIDS)—the sudden, unexpected death of previously healthy babies in which autopsy reveals no convincing cause of death.

The usual history is that the infant, whose age may range from 2 weeks to 2 years, was put to bed and died peacefully within the next 3–4 hours. This syndrome is not rare. A recent estimate placed the annual mortality in the United States as high as 10,000. Postmortem findings include some degree of cyanosis, petechial hemorrhages in the pericardium and lungs, and histologic evidence of diffuse, severe congestion with scattered hemorrhages and edema in the latter organs. Attempts to incriminate an infectious agent have so far failed.

In 1954 Dr. A. M. Barrett, an English pathologist, made the ingenious suggestion that these deaths might be related to a hypersensitivity reaction in the lungs to food aspirated during sleep. Subsequently he and a team of workers examined the possibility that cow's milk was the causal allergen, a notion sustained by knowledge of the relatively high incidence of allergy to cow's milk among bottle-fed babies, and its general manifestation following ingestion of this material. The latter evidence suggested the risk of a severe anaphylactic reaction if milk gained access to the lungs of highly hypersensitive individuals since, in man, as in the guinea pig, the lung is a "shock organ" in this type of response.

A variety of clinical observations and experimental findings have provided strong support for this explanation of crib death, which assigns what Dr. R. R. A. Coombs of the University of Cambridge, England, has referred to as a "Frankenstein role" to cow's milk. These include (1) The almost exclusive occurrence of crib death among bottle-fed babies. (2) The findings that whereas breast-fed babies rarely have significant titers of antibody against cow's milk proteins, bottle-fed infants develop antibodies as early as the second week postpartum, presumably as a result of the absorption of small amounts of the immunogenic proteins in an active, essentially undegraded form. Of course these antibodies, which are detectable by a hemagglutination technique, are not the mediators of immediate or anaphylactic-type sensitization, though their presence is indicative of the possibility of this type of sensitization. IgE is responsible for this. This immunoglobulin is normally bound to receptors on mast cells and basophils and its reaction with antigen causes the release from these cells of a variety of pharmacologic mediators, including histamine, SRS (slow reacting substance), and serotonin, which affect capillary vasodilation and permeability and smooth muscle contraction. (3) Young guinea pigs, sensitized against cow's milk either by inoculation or by feeding, respond to inhalation of cow's milk or material from the stomachs of bottle-fed babies by anaphylactic reactions of extreme violence bearing no resemblance to the apparently quiet demise of victims of crib death. When cow's milk was introduced into the tracheas of specifically sensitized guinea pigs that had been lightly anesthetized to simulate sleeping babies, however, both the manner of their deaths and the postmortem findings resembled those associated with crib death. (4) The presence of milk proteins has been demonstrated in the lungs of a high proportion of crib death victims. There is also a case on record of sudden death following inhalation of a small amount of milk by a sensitized child.

In view of the weight of circumstantial evidence sustaining the hypothesis that crib death is caused by anaphylactic reactivity to cow's milk, it is surprising that it has not gained wider acceptance. Evidence of the occurrence of crib death in a few exclusively breast-fed babies does not necessarily refute it, for these could be rare examples of anaphylactic-type sensitization to autoantigens (see page 68). To clinch the matter, it is obviously necessary to establish that an anaphylactic reaction has indeed occurred in its putative victims. The unavoidable delay between the time of death and postmortem examination is the problem here.

Finally, additional clinical observations concerning crib death, which have yet to be explained, include the preponderance of affected males and the higher incidence of the disease among Negroes than among Caucasians.

THE NEGLECTED CELLULAR COMPONENT OF MILK
AND ITS POSSIBLE SIGNIFICANCE

Histologists have long been aware that, in addition to epithelial cells and their disintegration products, leukocytes of various types are usually present in exocrine secretions. This holds true for saliva and urine and for the glandular secretions associated with the mucous membranes of the trachea and intestine. In view of the enormous aggregate surface area of the alveolar and ductal epithelium of the mammary gland during lactation, one might anticipate that some leukocytes would normally be present as well as effete epithelial cells in both colostrum and milk. It is well established that hypertrophy of the secretory epithelium of the mammary gland during pregnancy is accompanied by a conspicuous infiltration of the interstitial tissue by mononuclear cells of the lymphocytic series and that, soon after parturition, as the secretion of colostrum gives way to that of milk, the intensity of this cellular infiltration gradually decreases. In addition to cell fragments, colostrum contains large, nucleate cells with fat droplets in their cytoplasm, usually described as colostrum corpuscles. Although many early workers regarded these as transformed epithelial cells, others correctly identified them as leukocytic elements of hematogenous origin that had escaped from the connective tissue, traversed the epithelium, and entered the glandular lumen where they phagocytosed fat droplets.

From the beginning of this century, as the dairy industry came under the surveillance of Public Health Authorities, attention was focused upon the identity of the precursors and the prevalence of these cells in milk. This was prompted by the notion that, at least when present in large numbers, they must be indicative of pathologic conditions in the udder, notably mastitis. Reflective of this not unreasonable preoccupation is the title of a paper published in 1914 by R. S. Breed—"The sanitary significance of body cells in milk." The results of about 50 years' study are very inconsistent because of divergent opinions on the identity of these cells. There is no doubt, however, that bovine colostrum as well as milk normally contains considerable numbers of cells. Although actual counts vary within wide limits, the average is of the order of $0.5–1 \times 10^6$/ml. The count varies widely from day to day in milk drawn from the same cow, and even from different quarters of her udder. Furthermore, milk drawn later in milking usually contains more cells than milk drawn earlier. It is also generally recognized that cell counts considerably exceeding 1×10^6 per milliliter are not necessarily indicative of a diseased udder. In addition to epithelial cells, neutrophil polymorphonuclear cells, and both large and small lymphocytes are present, usually in approximately equal numbers. Eosinophils are rarely present.

In rats, too, leukocytes of hematogeneous origin participate in lactation and are normal components of milk (see Fig. 14-1). In 1926 Dr. V. E. Emmel and his co-workers at the University of Illinois College of Medicine presented evidence that active nursing is accompanied by a profound leukopenia in which the peripheral leukocyte count may fall by 50% or more. Quantitative histologic studies indicated an increased passage of lymphocytes into the glandular alveoli in association with the decrease of these cells from the circulation. Unfortunately, these workers provided no quantitative data on the cellular content of rat's milk. In the authors' laboratory it has been found that rat's milk normally contains $2–15 \times 10^6$ leukocytes per milliliter. Lipid-laden macrophages constitute approximately 75%; lymphocytes (both small and large) constitute about 23%; and polymorphonuclear lymphocytes, 2%.

In man the cellular component of colostrum and milk is just beginning to receive its long overdue consideration. Leukocytes are regular constituents of this exosecretion at concentrations that bear some resemblance to those of the blood. The leukocyte concentration of colostrum ranges from $1.5–4.0 \times 10^6$ per milliliter, and comprises primarily macrophages with a significant proportion of lymphocytes, while that of milk is of the order of 1.5×10^6 per milliliter. About 90% of colostral leukocytes are mononuclear cells, whereas in milk about 65% belong to this category.

According to a recent report, human milk contains T and B lymphocytes in approximately equal proportions and, on the basis of in vitro tests, their functional capacity is inferior to their counterparts in peripheral

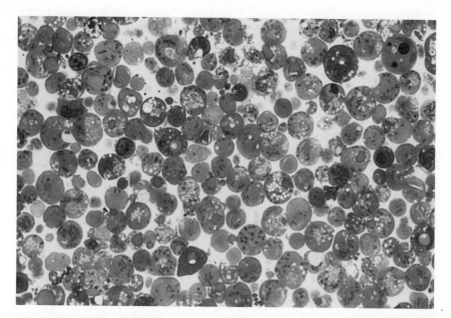

Fig. 14-1. Thin section through concentrated suspension of cells obtained from rat's milk. Note the abundant macrophages or milk 'corpuscles' with numerous lipid droplets in their cytoplasm. A few polymorphonuclear leukocytes and lymphocytes can also be identified.

blood. Colostral lymphocytes undergo blastoid transformation *in vitro* following exposure to phytohemagglutinin and also after exposure to such specific antigens as tetanus toxoid and penicillin. The macrophages attach to glass, display amoeboid movement, and phagocytose particulate material. Furthermore, when confronted by certain antigens *in vitro,* colostral leukocytes display the phenomenon of "migration inhibition," indicative of their ability to express delayed hypersensitivity reactivities acquired by the donor.

Comparison of the *in vitro* synthesis of proteins by human peripheral blood leukocytes on the one hand and by colostrum cells from the same donor on the other hand has shown that whereas the former synthesized IgA, IgM, β_{1c}/β_{1a}, and (less frequently) IgG, colostral cells synthesized IgA, β_{1c}/β_{1a}, and a protein specific to colostrum.

Apart from fulfilling a possible nutritive role, as suggested by some of the early workers, the recent findings on human colostral cells raise the possibility that colostral leukocytes may protect the breast against invading microorganisms. This they may do by phagocytosis as well as by release of IgA-type antibodies and nonspecific antimicrobial agents. It is also conceivable that "peripheral sensitization" may occur. Following encounter by an antigen-sensitive lymphocyte with a pathogen in the lumen of an alveolus or duct, the "primed" cell may reenter the interstitial tissue, establish itself in a regional lymph node, and generate a clone of responding cells.

EVIDENCE OF NATURAL TRANSPLANTATION OF
LEUKOCYTES DURING SUCKLING IN RATS

In the course of an analysis of the influence of interstrain pregnancies on the reactivity of adult Fischer strain rats to skin allografts from their infant (Fischer × DA) F_1 progeny, the present authors, in a collaborative study with Dr. Judith Head, observed that a small proportion of the normal babies, whose siblings had donated skin grafts to their lactating mothers when they were 5 days old, developed spreading exfoliative lesions of their perianal and abdominal skin when they were about 2 weeks old. Occasionally the skin of the dorsum was involved. No affected animal ever appeared sick or displayed growth retardation, however, and its skin usually became normal within several weeks. The fur of a small proportion of the affected individuals, as it subsequently grew, was sparse and conspicuously ruffled and remained so for many weeks. Skin lesions of this type were not observed in litters born of and raised by similar but non-grafted mothers. Since similar skin lesions are familiar harbingers of runt or graft-versus-host disease in infant rats, it occurred to us that specifically immune lymphocytes from the postpartum-sensitized mothers might have gained access to the tissues of their sucklings via the milk and initiated moderate runt disease. Transfer of insufficient numbers of putative attacking cells could explain the recovery of affected individuals.

Encouraged by these unexpected and still enigmatic findings, we have employed some familiar basic principles of transplantation immunology to determine whether maternal leukocytes normally gain access to the tissues of suckling rats via the milk.

Three groups of neonatal Fischer rats were, respectively, subjected to the following treatments: .

Group A (controls) were left with and raised by their normal Fischer mothers.

Group B were immediately transferred to lactating Lewis strain foster mothers *before* they had received any milk from their natural mothers.

Group C were allowed to suckle from their Fischer mothers for 24 hours, after which they too were transferred to Lewis foster mothers.

When these three groups of infants were 21 days old, they were challenged with skin allografts from Lewis donors to determine whether the reactivity of those in the experimental groups (B and C) differed from that of the controls as a consequence of ingesting milk from the alien Lewis mothers. Accelerated rejection would be indicative of prior sensitization (or less likely of nonspecific stimulation of their immunologic response machinery). Delayed rejection would express the induction of tolerance or less likely of immunologic enhancement. Either of these altered modalities of response would surely turn upon prior passage, through the wall of the digestive tract, of viable, milk-borne, maternal cells into the tissuse of the infants under study.

The results were clear-cut: The median survival time (MST) of the grafts on the "control" Fischer infants nursed throughout by their natural Fischer mothers was 10.2 ± 0.6 days, and none of these grafts lived longer than 13 days. Group C animals—i.e., those suckled by Lewis mothers after 24 hours' sustenance by their Fischer mothers—rejected their test grafts in an *accelerated* manner, the MST being 6.8 ± 1.5 days. The simplest and most likely explanation of this observation is that, as a result of their initial period of suckling on Fischer mothers, these animals received a "transfusion" of syngeneic adult, immunocompetent cells. During their subsequent foster nursing by Lewis strain mothers, when these infants absorbed allogeneic Lewis leukocytes from the milk, the previously acquired and now established adult Fischer immunocytes responded to the cellular antigen, generating a population of effector cells that made a significant contribution to the hyperreactivity to Lewis skin allografts expressed by these animals.

Finally the group B animals, whose sole source of milk had been Lewis mothers, displayed a significant degree of *hyporeactivity* to their test grafts. The MST of these grafts was 12.0 ± 1.4 days and more important a few grafts survived for as long as 26 days, presumably expressing the existence of incomplete tolerance of the antigens concerned. This particular donor-host strain combination is particularly favorable for tolerance induction studies since the intravenous inoculation of neonatal Fischer hosts with as few as 0.25×10^6 lymphomyeloid cells from an adult Lewis donor induces a significant degree of tolerance in respect of Lewis test skin grafts transplanted to them 50 days later.

Further circumstantial evidence of the natural transmission of viable leukocytes via the milk was afforded by the observation that about 30% of the group B infants developed and succumbed to runt disease. It is reasonable to believe that the induction of tolerance of the absorbed allogeneic cells contributed to their susceptibility. By contrast, none of the group C infants developed the disease, probably because of destruction or inactivation of the potentially harmful alien cells by the milk-transferred adult Fischer immunocompetent cells—i.e., the animals were adoptively immunized. Also no Fischer offspring suckled solely on a (Fischer × Lewis)F_1 mother died.

Suckling DA babies on Fischer mothers proved to have little effect on their reactivity to subsequent test grafts of Fischer skin and none of them developed graft-versus-host disease. Here, no doubt because of the magnitude of the immunogenetic disparity involved, the MST of control skin grafts was only 6.6 ± 1.1 days so that the test system was probably not sufficiently sensitive to reveal weak sensitization. Furthermore, with this strain combination the cell dosage requirements for the induction of tolerance are much higher than are likely to be met by natural "inoculation" of cells via the milk.

We are currently trying to increase the leukocyte concentration of rat breast milk in the hope of augmenting the number of cells transferred to infants by suckling. It has been found that the milk of Fischer females who have gestated and raised several allogeneic (Fischer × DA)F$_1$ hybrid litters contains no more leukocytes than the milk of Fischer females who have raised several syngeneic litters. However, Fischer females who have rejected allografts of DA skin prior to pregnancy by Fischer males have approximately twice as many leukocytes in their milk as previously ungrafted mothers throughout lactation. Despite this leukocytosis in the milk of previously allografted females, which persists for approximately 4 months, their peripheral blood leukocyte counts remained within normal limits. Intravenous injection of lactating Fischer females with *Bordatella pertussis* induces a striking leukocytosis in the peripheral blood but only rather erratically is the leukocyte concentration of their milk elevated. Indeed, in some subjects this treatment appeared to reduce the leukocyte population of the milk. It is obvious that the factors, both internal and external, that control both the leukocyte concentration in milk and the immunological status of its lymphocyte moiety are far less well understood than the mechanisms controlling the concentration and types of humoral antibodies present in this mammary gland exosecretion.

CONCLUSIONS

Various means have evolved, depending on the species, of providing an important endowment of ready-made maternal humoral antibodies to tide the newborn mammal over the critical first few weeks as it builds up its own repertoire of immunologic experience. Probably the risk of runt disease has been an important factor precluding the evolution of a similar means of providing a beneficial maternal endowment of *cellular* immunities. At least in man, however, we cannot entirely exclude the possibility that placental porosity to lymphocytes may confer some transient advantage upon the baby, especially if sensitized or effector cells release informational molecules such as Dr. H. S. Lawrence's "transfer factor," which might have an amplifying effect. This slight advantage may exact its price, however, for even if the number of cells transferred from mother to fetus is small, and they are soon destroyed by host reactivity, they might initiate transient, subclinical GVH reactions with overt consequences. Studies in mice have shown that GVH reactivity may result in a high incidence of lymphomas, probably because of its ability to unmask and activate normally latent and undemonstrable oncogenic viruses. The relatively high incidence of lymphomas in children might also be attributable in part to GVH reactivity on the part of cells of maternal origin.

The considerations that apply to maternal lymphocytes transmitted across the placenta would also apply to similar cells gaining access to the neonate's tissues via the milk, as in the rat. One possible protective role that milk-borne leukocytes may play in human infants is under current investigation. A significant toll of human babies is taken by a disease known as necrotizing enterocolitis. This disease is not infrequently encountered in neonatal and very young infants. The clinical symptoms are abdominal distention, diarrhea, and blood in the feces. Pathologic findings are breakdown in the integrity of the epithelium of the gastrointestinal tract and invasion of the wall of the gut by gas-forming microorganisms and their subsequent dissemination. Predisposing etiologic factors, which may act singly or in combination, appear to be prematurity, transient asphyxia, disturbance of the splanchnic circulation, as a consequence of blood transfusion via the umbilical vein, infection, and feeding. Dr. J. Pitt and her colleagues at Columbia-Presbyterian Hospital in New York have shown that a faithful model of this disease is procurable in newborn rats by subjecting them to hypoxia and exposing them to enteric pathogens. All succumb to the disease within a few days if formula-fed but not if they are breast-fed. Various findings indicated that the presence of viable macrophages in the feed, either from the milk or from the blood or peritoneal exudates, was essential for protection. Killing of bacterial pathogens by these cells appeared to be the basis of the protection.

There are two implications of the capacity of at least some infant animals to absorb lymphocytes in a viable form from their milk that may be of significance for the experimental immunologist.

1. This represents an equipping of an immunologically immature host with a variable number of mature, antigen-reactive cells, i.e., a form of *adoptive immunization*. With some donor-host strain combinations this may be a factor contributing to the difficulty of inducing tolerance of alloantigens by neonatal injection of living donor cells or to the variability in results obtained with more favorable strain combinations. Indeed this reasoning has been validated by foster-nursing homozygous infants from birth onward by appropriate F_1 hybrid females facilitating tolerogenesis of transplantation alloantigens (See Fig. 14-2).

2. Milk may be a neglected but important source of T lymphocytes in

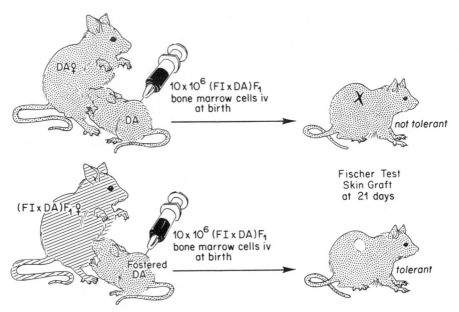

Fig. 14-2. Illustrating the influence of the source of the milk cells an infant rat receives on the facility with which it can be rendered tolerant of tissue allografts by neonatal intravenous injection of living allogeneic cells. Much higher doses of (FI × DA)F$_1$ hybrid bone marrow cells must be injected into neonatal DA hosts to induce tolerance of subsequent skin allografts from FI donors if they suckle on their own DA mothers than if they are foster-nursed by (FI × DA)F$_1$ mothers. For example, an inoculum of 10 × 10^6 cells is usually effective in the latter situation but not in the former.

both neonatally thymectomized mice as well as in "nude" mice in which the thymus is congenitally absent.

The idea that a mother or a wet nurse can influence an infant's health both adversely as well as favorably through the milk has a long history. For example, in his *Anatomy of Melancholy* (1621) Robert Burton wrote "From a Childs nativity, the first ill accident that can likely befall him in this kind, is a bad nurse. . . ." Some of the observations considered in this chapter afford it a cellular immune basis.

REFERENCES

Beer, A. E., and Billingham, R. E. 1973. "Maternally acquired runt disease." *Science* **179**:240–243.

Beer, A. E., Billingham, R. E., and Head, J. 1974. "The immunological significance of the mammary gland." *J. Invest. Dermatol.* **63**:65–74.

Billingham, R. E., Defendi, V., Silvers, W. K., and Steinmuller, D. 1962. "Quantitative studies on induction of tolerance of skin homografts and on runt disease in neonatal rats." *J. Nat. Can. Inst.* **28**:365–435.

Brambell, F. W. R. 1970. *The transmission of passive immunity from mother to young.* American Elsevier, New York.

Caroli, J., and Bessis, M. 1947. "Immunisation de la mère par le foetus chez la jument mulassière. Son rôle dans l'ictère grave du muleton." *C. r. Séanc. Soc. Biol.* **141**:386–387.

Coombs, R. 1963. "An experimental model for cot deaths." In *Sudden death in infants* (R. J. Wedgwood and E. P. Benditt, ed.). National Institute of Child Health and Human Development. Bethesda, Md. Public Health Service Publication No. 1412, pp. 55–74.

Diaz-Jouanen, E. P., and Williams, R. C. 1974. "T and B cells in human colostrum." *Clin. Res.* **22**:416A.

Dixon, F. J., Weigle, W. O., and Vazquez, J. J. 1961. "Metabolism and mammary secretion of serum proteins in the cow." *Lab. Invest.* **10**:216–237.

Emmel, V. E., Weatherford, H. L., and Streicher, M. H. 1926. "Leucocytes and lactation." *Am. J. Anatomy* **38**:1–39.

Hanson, L. A., and Winberg, J. 1972. "Breast milk and defense against infection in the newborn." *Arch. Dis. Child.* **47**:845–847.

Holm, G. C. 1934. "The types of leucocytes in market milk as related to bovine mastitis." *J. Am. Vet. Med. Assn.* **35**:735–747.

Mohr, J. A., Leu, R., and Mabry, W. 1970. "Colostral leucocytes." *J. Surg. Oncol.* **2**:163–167.

Morse, S. I. 1965. "Studies on lymphocytosis induced in mice by *Bordetella pertussis.*" *J. Exp. Med.* **121**:49–68.

Murillo, G. J. 1971. "Synthesis of secretory IgA by human colostral cells." *South. Med. J.* **64**:1333–1337.

Palm, J. 1970. "Maternal-fetal interactions and histocompatibility antigen polymorphisms." *Transpl. Proc.* **2**:162–173.

Parish, W. E., Barrett, A. M., Coombs, R. R. A., Gunther, M., and Camps, F. E. 1960. "Hypersensitivity to milk and sudden death in infancy." *Lancet* **ii**:1106–1110.

Pitt, J., Barlow, B., Heird, W. C., and Santulli, T. V. 1974. "Macrophages and protective action of breast milk in necrotizing enterocolitis." *Pediat. Res.* **8**:384.

Schwartz, R. S. 1972. "Immuoregulation, oncogenic viruses, and malignant lymphomas." *Lancet* i:1266–1269.

Smith, C. W., and Goldman, A. S. 1968. "The cells of human colostrum. *In vitro* studies of morphology and functions." *Pediat. Res.* 2:103–109.

Torma, M. J., Delemos, R. A., Rogers, J. R., and Diserens, H. W. 1973. "Necrotizing enterocolitis in infants." *Am. J. Surg.* 126:758–761.

Touloukian, R. J., Posch, J. N., and Spencer, R. 1972. "The pathogenesis of ischemic gastroenterocolitis of the neonate: selective gut mucosal ischemia in asphyxiated neonatal piglets." *J. Pediat. Surg.* 7:194–205.

Vahlquist, B. 1958. "The transfer of antibodies from mother to offspring. *Adv. Pediat.* 10:305–338.

Valdes-Dapena, M. 1963. "Serum proteins, viral isolation, antibodies to milk, and epidemiologic factors in sudden death." In *Sudden death in infants* (R. J. Wedgwood and E. P. Benditt, ed.). National Institute of Child Health and Human Development. Bethesda, Md. Public Health Service Publication No. 1412, pp. 75–91.

Varrier-Jones, P. C. 1924. "The cellular content of milk: variations met with under physiological and pathological conditions." *Lancet* ii:537–543.

Chapter 15

Histocompatibility Gene Polymorphisms and Maternal-Fetal Interactions

Although there are no factual grounds for supposing that antigenic diversity is anything but an unfortunate consequence of constitutional differences between individuals of a species, yet one is under some obligation to rack one's brains for evidence of any good it might conceivably do. Only thus can antigenic polymorphism be made genetically respectable.—P. B. Medawar, 1953.

Over the last few years considerable progress appears to have been made in unraveling the biological significance of histocompatibility antigens and so explaining why it has been advantageous for mammals, and indeed other vertebrates, to possess that extreme degree of genetic diversity expressed at the level of the cell surface structures, which is revealed by transplantation. In certain experimental animals, notably in mice, rats, and guinea pigs, very close associations have now been shown to exist between histocompatibility alleles at the major histocompatibility complex, the capacity to react against certain synthetic branched-chain polypeptides and susceptibility to oncogenic viruses. In man, too, a formidable body of unequivocal evidence has now been amassed associating susceptibility to certain malignant and other diseases with some HL-A locus specificities.

Knowledge of (1) the very considerable polymorphism of the major histocompatability systems in different species, (2) the expression of their products on the plasma membranes of spermatozoa and of cells of both preimplantation and postimplantation embryos, and (3) the fact that alterations of the maternal immune response do occur in response to fetal antigens raised several questions. What mechanism(s) allows allogeneic fetuses to escape maternal immunologic attack? Does this membrane antigen polymorphism lead to selective processes that might operate (1) at fertilization, (2) during the process of nidation, and (3) through interactions at the tissue or cellular level (including mutual cellular exchanges) between the fetus and its mother? The purpose of this chapter is to review some of the evidence and concepts that bear upon this important topic.

217

DEPARTURES FROM EXPECTED MENDELIAN
SEGREGATION RATIOS IN EXPERIMENTAL ANIMALS

When animals of two different inbred strains are mated, producing F_1 hybrid embryos that confront their mothers with alien, paternally inherited histocompatibility antigens, the litters tend to be larger and healthier than those resulting from intrastrain matings, due, so it is commonly asserted, to heterosis or hybrid vigor. Such observations afford no proof, however, that hybrids enjoy any particular advantage over genetically compatible offspring from conception to birth. To test this hypothesis entails comparison of the relative abilities of the two types of embryo to thrive in the same uterine milieu. The experimental approach requires animals of two different inbred strains differing with respect to histocompatibility alleles that can be identified. Appropriate matings can then be set up to produce segregated populations of R_2 backcross or F_2 generations that can be tested to find out whether the H genotypes are present in the expected Mendelian ratios. For example, if we have two strains of mice that differ with respect to alleles at the H-2 locus, one H-2^a/H-2^a and the other H-2^k/H-2^k, we would expect to find H-2^a/H-2^a, H-2^a/H-2^k, and H-2^k/H-2^k individuals present in the ratio 1:2:1 in the F_2 generation. Alternatively, if we mate H-2^a/H-2^k mice with H-2^a/H-2^a mice to produce a backcross population, we should expect to find the genotypes H-2^a/H-2^a and H-2^a/H-2^k in equal proportions. Significant deviations from these expected ratios would be suggestive of the operation of some kind of prenatal selective factor. An alternative and more tedious approach that we have been pursuing in the rat is to transfer fertilized eggs in equal numbers from homozygous allogeneic donors and from syngeneic donors to homozygous, pseudopregnant females. In one experiment, this has entailed the insertion of eggs from Fischer females mated with males of this strain and eggs from DA females mated with DA males into the uteri of FI females. Here the coat color phenotypes of the progeny are directly indicative of their genotypes.

Experiments of the former type have been performed by various investigators and the findings indicate that conceptuses that are disparate with their mothers at certain histocompatibility loci enjoy a slight selective advantage over conceptuses that are compatible with their mothers at these loci.

Hull carried out an experiment with mice of the C57BL/10 (H-3^a/H-3^a) strain and the congenic resistant strain B10.LP, which differs from the former only with respect to a chromosomal segment bearing a different allele (H-3^b/H-3^b) at the relatively minor H-3 locus. He found that when H-3^a/H-3^b males were backcrossed to either H-3^a/H-3^a or H-3^b/H-3^b females, significantly fewer than the expected 50% of the progeny were homozygous at this locus—i.e., there was an *excess* of *heterozygotes*. Furthermore, this deficiency in homozygotes was only observable among the offspring of later (i.e., third and fourth) litters from H-3^a/H-3^a mothers and only among the males from H-3^b/H-3^b females. When reciprocal matings were set up, using F$_1$ hybrid mothers and homozygous fathers, the expected segregation ratios were obtained. Since there were no significant differences in the weights at birth or at weaning between the homozygotes and heterozygotes born of homozygous mothers, these interesting findings suggest that if differential mortality is associated with this apparent "auto-incompatibility," it may take place soon after conception and after this critical stage the survivors develop normally. Hull's finding that, with one of the crosses he tested, deficient segregation ratios occurred only among the third and fourth litters suggested that maternal sensitization to the alien tissue antigen was an important factor in conferring a selective advantage upon the heterozygotes. It is unfortunate that this hypothesis was not tested by specifically sensitizing the homozygous females against the alien antigen of their F$_1$ hybrid consorts before mating.

In rats, two independent studies have furnished strong evidence of selective pressures that assured the survival of excess numbers of heterozygotes. In 1966, working at the University of Edinburgh, Drs. Michie and Anderson discovered a very striking example of heterozygote advantage during the course of investigating the failure of 72 generations of brother × sister matings of Wistar rats to produce an isohistogenic strain—i.e., a strain whose members would consistently accept grafts of each others' skin. Their analysis revealed that the majority of the surviving rats were *heterozygotes*, resulting from an intense selection against individuals that were homozygous for genes at an undefined H locus. These workers were able to select and breed some of the few surviving progeny of one homozygote class, producing an isohistogenic strain, but they failed to recover the second class of homozygote. Since litter-size data suggested that the selective elimination of the homozygotes took place *before* implantation of the blastocysts, Michie and Anderson postulated that if the allelic histocompatibility genes concerned were g$_1$ and g$_2$ and the survival value of the heterozygous individuals was superior to that of either homozygote, this situation might result from *selective fertilization,* i.e., by g$_1$ sperm uniting preferentially with g$_2$ eggs and g$_2$ sperm, with g$_1$ eggs. Subsequent evidence that histocompatibility determinants are expressed by spermatozoa in mice, rats, hamsters, and man is consonant with this interesting explanation.

Working with the same stock of rats, the late Dr. Joy Palm, at the Wistar Institute, has confirmed Michie and Anderson's observations and shown, in addition, that segregation at the major Ag-B locus is not responsible for the phenomenon. In an extensive, long-term study of the Ag-B locus phenotypes of the backcross progeny of 12 different inbred rat strain combinations she has found that, in all but 2 strain combinations, there is a consistent and statistically significant excess of Ag-B locus *heterozygotes*. Furthermore, the excess of Ag-B heterozygotes was more striking among males than females, reflecting greater vulnerability of male than female homozygotes.

The results of a particularly careful study of the BN and DA strain backcrosses indicated that the deficiency of Ag-B compatible progeny resulted from an *active reduction* in this class rather than from a nonspecific selective advantage enjoyed by the Ag-B heterozygotes (see Fig. 15.1). This reduction of the expected numbers of Ag-B compatible offspring could occur either prenatally or postnatally, depending on the genetics of the particular mating. With some of the strain combinations tested the post-

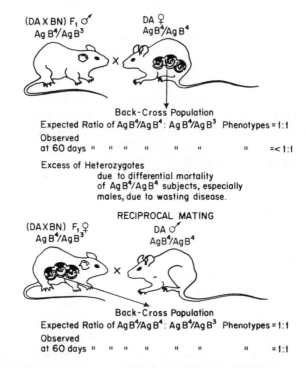

Fig. 15-1. Illustrating the unexpected, different Ag-B locus segregation ratios in reciprocal backcross matings obtained by Dr. Joy Palm with rats of the DA(Ag-B⁴) and BN(Ag-B³) strains. Apart from differing at the Ag-B locus, these strains also differ at other histocompatibility loci. When DA females were mated to (BN × DA)F₁ males, there was an excess of Ag-B heterozygotes among the progeny—i.e., of animals that are incompatible with their mothers at this locus. Careful observations revealed that this unexpected departure from the expected 1:1 ratio resulted from a selective mortality rate among infants that were compatible with their mothers at the Ag-B locus, probably attributable to runt or graft-versus-host disease. This disease affected twice as many Ag-B homozygotes as heterozygotes, and males were more susceptible than females (see page 172).

natal reduction of the Ag-B compatible class of progeny was the outcome of a wasting disease having all the hallmarks of GVH or runt disease, including retarded growth, abnormalities of the skin, and (in extreme cases) involution of lymphoid tissue. The severity of these symptoms, their time of onset, and death, if it occurred, was found to be related to parity, the onset being progressively earlier in later litters.

When matings of rat strains that were compatible at the Ag-B locus but differed at other genetic loci were set up, of eight different combinations tested, only one produced live offspring and all of these succumbed to the wasting syndrome before weaning. Subsequent fertility tests on the partners in these unproductive matings—involving mating with either syngeneic or Ag-B incompatible rats—confirmed their fertile status and sustained the important conclusion that when Ag-B locus incompatibility is lacking, reproductive performance is greatly curtailed. It will be interesting to determine whether, with such strain combinations, induction of tolerance in the females with regard to the tissue alloantigens of their future mates will render them fertile.

Sustaining Palm's tentative conclusion that this selective elimination of homozygotes, which may take place either prenatally or postnatally, results from an immune response on the part of the mother against some non-Ag-B histocompatibility antigen (or differentiation antigen) are the following observations: (1) Normal segregation ratios occur among the progeny of F_1 hybrid females backcrossed to parental strain males. Under this circumstance, of course, all the females are genetically tolerant of and so incapable of reacting against all their offspring's transplantation antigens. (2) A wasting syndrome similar to that resulting from GVH reactivity occurred among the depressed Ag-B compatible class. (3) The severity of this disease increased with increasing parity of the mother.

Individuals that are heterozygous at the Ag-B locus, and so differ from their Ag-B homozygous mothers with respect to antigens determined by one Ag-B allele, likewise differ from their mothers at non-Ag-B histocompatibility loci, including one or more that are probably responsible for their susceptibility to the postulated incompatibility reactions. Thus, in this particular genetic context, incompatibility with its mother at the Ag-B locus seems to confer protection upon the fetus against the development and/or consequences of immunological reactivity on the part of the mother against antigens determined by other loci.

Palm's observation that, in different strain combinations where deficiencies of the expected numbers of Ag-B compatible progeny were observed, there was an excess of albino offspring—i.e., a deficiency of the Cc heterozygotes suggested that the genetic locus determining one antigen responsible for the loss of perinatal rats might be linked to the albino locus. As Palm pointed out, this clear-cut, selective advantage of Ag-B heterozygotes in laboratory populations of rats might well reflect an important, naturally occurring phenomenon among wild populations that would influence the degree of polymorphism at the Ag-B locus.

ALLOANTIGENS AND SEGREGATION RATIOS IN MAN

In man the remarkable degree of variability of the HL-A system, coupled with its importance for histocompatibility and its possible significance with respect to the control of the immune system and consequent disease associations, emphasizes the question of how this polymorphism is maintained by selective forces, if differential selection is involved. Obviously departures from the expected Mendelian segregation of HL-A antigens in families would constitute the simplest and most direct evidence for selection. However, these would only measure selection due to viability differentials associated with different HL-A phenotypes and provide no information on possible fertility differentials. So far, data on the segregation of single HL-A antigens in backcrosses and intercrosses have provided no indications of departure from expected Mendelian ratios. Study of the segregation of single HL-A antigens would not reveal disturbances associated with particular haplotypes however, and it is unlikely that it would reveal incompatibility selection due to the effects of maternal antibody on the fetuses. Although more complex tests for revealing deviation from expected Mendelian segregation without identifying particular antigens have been devised and employed, these, too, have failed to yield evidence of significant departures from expectation in the absence of selection.

The relatively high incidence of fetal-maternal stimulation with respect to HL-A antigens and, of course, the occurrence of natural examples of maternally induced GVH disease pose the question whether these antigens may not be associated with significant incompatibility selection. This is a process that generally acts *against* polymorphism since it leads to heterozygote disadvantage. Incompatibility selection does occur in the case of hemolytic disease of the newborn, due to antigens of the Rh system and very rarely to antigens of the ABO blood groups (see Chapter 11). These latter antigens are now recognized to be important determinants of histocompatibility and consequently it is pertinent to ask whether there is any evidence of ABO interaction between mother and child earlier in pregnancy. On an immunological basis one can distinguish between "compatible" and "incompatible" marriages with respect to these antigens. The former are those in which the mother's blood contains only those anti-A or anti-B antibodies for which her children lack the corresponding antigens. Incompatible marriages are those in which children may be produced whose antigens can be attacked by the mother's antibodies.

Although surveys have been made of the outcome of ABO incompatible pregnancies, the results have been inconsistent. In some surveys evidence of a deficiency of children with incompatible genotypes was obtained, leading to the conclusion that prenatal mortality was responsible for the loss of such children. In a study of families in Japan, Matsunaga found that in the compatible matings of A women to O men the proportion of A and O children was in accordance with expectation from the allele frequences in the population. In the reciprocal incompatible matings of O women to A men, however, there was a deficiency of A children. This difference in the outcome of the reciprocal matings appeared to result from the loss of incompatible fetuses in O women. Since the total stillbirth rates in children in these two reciprocal matings were similar, it was postulated that early spontaneous abortions were responsible for the loss of incompatible A fetuses. Indeed the frequency of abortions in the A × O matings was less than in the O × A matings. Later studies in Japan by Matsunaga and his associates have given no evidence for extensive fetal loss in ABO incompatible pregnancies. Obviously additional studies are required to clarify this situation.

As far as the HL-A antigens are concerned, it is well established that HL-A antibodies do not, in general, exert any harmful effects on fetuses and there is no convincing evidence that a higher proportion of stillbirths or abortions is associated with maternal HL-A sensitization. A search has yet to be made, however, for fertility differences associated with different degrees of HL-A incompatibility between mother and offspring.

Another possible example of incompatibility selection in man pertains to the X-linked Xg^a erythrocyte antigen. Although the sex ratios of children from marriages of Xg(a+) × Xg(a+), Xg(a−) × Xg(a−), and Xg(a+) × Xg(a−) fall within the normal range, that from Xg(a−) × Xg(a+) is significantly higher than normal. This may be the result of an incompatibility reaction, often leading to fetal loss, on the part of Xg(a−) mothers against their Xg(a+) zygotes. The finding that the sex ratio is even higher in those children born after the first Xg(a+) daughter lends support to this hypothesis. Antibodies induced by the first Xg(a+) pregnancy might lead to the increased loss of subsequent female fetuses. Indeed, it has been suggested by Drs. Jackson, Mann, and Schull, who in 1969 made these observations, that Xg^a incompatibility may help to explain the lower frequency of female than male births in general.

In 1966 Clarke and Kirby postulated that some kind of immunological interaction between females and their histoincompatible fetuses might, contrary to expectation, actually *favor* the survival of such offspring and thus help maintain the complex histocompatibility polymorphisms found in mammals. Their thesis rested on evidence that in mice and other species both placental size and fetal size are affected by antigenic differences,

224 HISTOCOMPATIBILITY GENE POLYMORPHISMS

suggesting that fetuses that are unlike their mothers—i.e., confront the latter with foreign antigens—tend to be larger at birth and have an increased chance of survival. In a review of 1970 the late Dr. Kirby suggested that blastocysts which are genetically dissimilar to their mothers implant more readily than blastocysts which are genetically similar.

THE Y-LINKED ANTIGEN AND ITS POSSIBLE INFLUENCE ON THE SEX RATIO IN MAN

Although evidence that man has a Y-linked histocompatibility locus homologous to that present in mice and rats has only recently been forthcoming, assumption that he does has led to some interesting speculations and interpretations of human data. In 1962 Renkonen, Mäkelä and Lehtovaara presented statistical evidence suggesting that at least two factors affect the human sex ratio: (1) Children of a certain parity tend to be boys if all the preceding children in the family have been boys, and they tend to be girls if all the preceding children have been girls. (2) If these "unisexual" families exhibiting this tendency are excluded, the sex ratio is the lower, the greater the number of preceding male pregnancies. Thus, so it is reasoned, in these families male pregnancies render the couples less likely to have additional boys, possibly as a consequence of immunization of the mother against the Y antigen. The implication here, of course, is that the immunization would be harmful to subsequent conceptuses.

Kirby and his associates offered an explanation of the human sex ratio of 0.516, which turned upon the assumption that male zygotes are always slightly more antigenic to their mothers than female zygotes by virtue of the superimposition of their Y-linked antigen upon the otherwise statistically equivalent, autosomally determined, paternal endowment of transplantation antigens. Since the results of sexing abortuses in humans indicate a considerably higher sex ratio early in pregnancy than at birth and yet animal studies suggest a more or less equal number of male and female zygotes before implantation, these workers consider that more female blastocysts fail to implant than male blastocysts, the superior implantability of the latter revolving about possession of a Y antigen.

According to this reasoning, inbreeding should tend to lessen the differences at autosomal histocompatibility loci between zygotes and their mothers and accentuate the importance of the Y antigen at implantation. This leads to the prediction that consanguineous marriages should produce a higher proportion of males than nonconsanguineous marriages. Reanalysis of previous data obtained by one of these authors revealed that the sex ratio (0.55) in one group of isolated, first-cousin marriages in a normal, outbreeding society was, indeed, significantly higher than the national average. Unfortunately, although essentially similar data have been obtained independently by some investigators in various communities in the world, the plausibility of this thesis is compromised by other studies that have failed to produce corroborative evidence of disturbed sex ratios among the progeny of consanguineous marriages, particularly in "closed" or isolated communities.

Subsequently, in 1970, Kirby suggested that the Y antigen in man may influence the sex ratio by interaction with antigens of the ABO blood group system. Assuming that these antigens are expressed by the early blastocyst, if mother and zygote are compatible with respect to them (i.e., the mother has no ready-made isoantibodies capable of reacting with the zygote), the Y-linked antigen of the latter should play a more important selective role in procuring successful implantation of male blastocysts than when the zygotes are ABO incompatible with their mothers. Kirby cited sex ratio data in relation to blood group findings that lent some support to this premise. For example, AB mothers have significantly more male than female babies, and this high sex ratio is also found among group O babies born of O mothers or among B babies born of B mothers. An important exception, however, that awaits explanation is that the sex ratio in A babies born of A mothers is low. Finally, *ex hypothesi,* irrespective of the blood group of their mothers, O babies should have a high sex ratio, and this situation does appear to prevail in practice.

Although maternal-fetal blood group incompatibilities have been under suspicion as a cause of toxemia of pregnancy for about 75 years, careful studies appear to have exonerated the ABO and Rh blood group systems, and there are now reasonable grounds for the belief that organ-specific or histocompatibility antigens associated with the trophoblast play a leading role (see Chapter 8).

In 1970, two Finnish workers, Toivanen and Hirvanen, reported that the sex ratio in babies born to toxemic mothers is significantly elevated (i.e., 1.24). Furthermore, they have shown that this ratio increases with the severity of the disease as determined by daily urinary protein excretion or blood pressure. To explain these interesting findings the authors suggested that paternally inherited histocompatibility antigens in the placenta may potentiate the immunogenicity of those antigens that this organ shares in common with the kidney and that are believed by many workers to be responsible for toxemia. Male fetuses might be expected to be slightly more antigenic than female fetuses in initiating this disease on account of their immunogenic "edge" or advantage from the postulated possession of a Y-chromosome-dependent transplantation antigen.

Drs. Scott and Beer have recently reported some interesting clinical data indicating that male fetuses are almost exclusively responsible for Rh isoimmunization in first pregnancies. In Rh-negative women who have had no known abortions or blood transfusions the incidence of Rh sensitization in first pregnancies is very low—of the order of 0.4–2.0%. Sensitization in these women results either from fetal → maternal bleeding very early in gestation, so that the mother develops an effective immune response *before* parturition, or from the mother's prior sensitization during her own fetal life *in utero* as a consequence of the receipt of Rh-positive cells from her mother. Subsequent reexposure to the antigen many years later, as a consequence of gestating an Rh-positive fetus, might result in a "secondary response"—i.e., the rapid, reawakening of the original sensitivity.

In a study of 25 patients in this category who developed Rh antibody before delivering their first child, 21 had been gestated by Rh-positive mothers. Only two of these patients were of blood type O despite the fact that approximately 50% of the women in the local population were of type O. More striking was the observation that in all but two cases the infant that incited the sensitization was an ABO compatible, Rh-positive *male*. Previous investigators had also noted high sex ratios among sensitizing, first-born children.

Among the possible explanations suggested by Scott and Beer for these observations are (1) A Y-linked antigen might render male erythrocytes more strongly immunogenic than female red cells. (2) The placentas of male fetuses may facilitate a greater volume of fetal-maternal cell traffic than female placentas. Another possibility is that Rh antigens may be expressed sooner in development in male than in female fetuses.

THE Y ANTIGEN IN THE MOUSE AND ITS INFLUENCE ON THE SEX RATIO

Speculators that a postulated Y-linked alloantigen may influence the sex ratio in man should take heed of some interesting experiments that have been performed in C57BL/6 mice. These animals have a genetical background on which the Y antigen is not trivial—the median survival time of grafts of syngeneic male skin on females being about 27 days.

Dr. Anne McLaren of the University of Edinburgh carried out an analysis of the influence of the state of reactivity of C57 female mice to the Y antigen on their reproductive performance when mated with males of their own strain. She found that, irrespective of whether the mother-to-be had received no prior treatment (i.e., were controls), had been specifically presensitized to the Y antigen, or had been made tolerant of it, before mating with C57 males, the mean numbers and sex ratios of the resultant litters were closely similar. It is worth emphasizing that the sex ratio in the progeny of the controls, as in the experimental series, was essentially unity.

By far the most interesting experiments along these lines were reported on in 1971 by Drs. Lappé and Schalk of the University of California at Berkeley. These investigators studied the influence of splenectomy prior to sensitization of adult virgin females of the C57 and RIII strains against the Y antigen, on the sex ratio of the progeny after subsequent mating with syngeneic males. Sensitization was effected 'by grafting with skin followed, 28 days later, by subcutaneous inoculation of spleen cells from syngeneic male donors. Controls were provided by sham-splenectomized and subsequently immunized females and by splenectomized females inoculated with spleen cells from syngeneic *female* donors.

As McLaren has previously found, immunization of females whose spleens were intact had no influence on the sex ratio. Immunization subsequent to the removal of this organ, however, significantly increased the proportion of males born. Furthermore it was noted that the most strongly sensitized females (in terms of the survival times of their skin grafts from male donors) gave birth to litters with the highest sex ratios.

Since there is evidence that, in the mouse, the preimplantation sex ratio is near equality, the events underlying these interesting and important observations must occur during or after fertilization. Lappé and Schalk present additional data, pertaining to litter sizes, etc., which sustain their thesis that "preferential salvation" of male conceptuses which would normally fail to implant may explain these observations. Corpora lutea counts on primiparous C57 females indicated that up to 30% more eggs may be available (half of which would produce males) than actually implant.

Since the balanced sex ratio found in most mouse strains seems to be maintained despite the known occurrence of maternal immunization to the Y antigen during pregnancy, the authors postulated that a spleen-associated factor, probably enhancing or blocking antibodies, may play a role in maintaining the normal sex ratio of one. It is now well documented that the spleen is the principal source of enhancing or blocking antibodies which prolong the lives of allografts (see pages 45, 161). The idea is that these antibodies may, in some way, interfere with the expression of the cellular immune response and the latter would favor a differential fertility effect.

The empirical fact that allogeneic fetuses in general appear to enjoy an advantage over genetically compatible fetuses probably reflects the operation of this same principle. Indeed, in the light of Palm's observations, and our own findings on the increased numbers of allogeneic blastocysts that implant in the locally and specifically sensitized uterine horns of rats, a study of the phenotype ratio resulting from backcross matings of F_1 males to splenectomized normal and specifically sensitized parental strain females would appear to be a fruitful line of investigation.

MATERNAL ENVIRONMENTAL INFLUENCE ON EXPRESSION
OF ANTIGENICITY AND IMMUNOLOGIC
RESPONSIVENESS IN MICE

Geneticists have long been interested in the influence of the maternal environment on the developing fetus. The expression of a number of inherited congenital characteristics of the progeny has been found to be correlated with physiological variables of the mother, especially with her age. Two well-known examples relate to the guinea pig. First, in a strain of polydactylous animals the older the mothers, the higher the proportion of young born with the normal number of toes. The second example of a prenatal maternal influence on the phenotype of the young is manifested in the relative size of the white patches of the coat in a spotted strain, the white areas of the progeny becoming larger with increasing age of the mother.

The fact that no clear examples of a paternal influence exist is hardly surprising since the paternal contribution to the zygote, the sperm, consists almost entirely of chromosomal material in its head, and of very little else that might exert any extragenic effect. By contrast, the oocyte contains a great deal of extragenetic material in its cytoplasm. In addition, the mother supplies the uterine environment in which the fetus develops; and she also sustains it postpartum via the breast.

We have already discussed the transmission of maternal cells and gamma globulins which are incorporated into the fetus at least transiently and which might be considered to have some influence on its phenotype. On an experimental basis foster nursing was shown to influence the growth of transplantable leukemias in mice and to influence both resistance and sensitivity to X irradiation. The technique of ova transplantation was originally developed to investigate possible maternal intrauterine influences and an early finding, by Dr. A. M. Cloudman, was that tumors of the foster mother's genetic makeup grew progressively in, and eventually killed, recipients of the ova-transfer substrain and even their descendants, but not hosts of their strain of origin.

Over the last 10 years, Dr. Delta Uphoff of the National Cancer Institute has been carrying out some rather complicated but exceedingly interesting experiments on mice that indicate that the maternal environment, including the milk, can influence the phenotypic expression of both antigenicity and immunologic responsiveness in the progeny and *that these phenotypic alterations are permanent and vertically transmitted from mother to offspring for many generations.*

To detect and study these changes, Uphoff has employed three different kinds of experimental subjects:

1. *Reciprocal hybrid mice* produced by mating parents of two different inbred strains so that females of each strain are mated to a male of the opposite strain, producing for example both $(A♀ \times B♂)F_1$ hybrids and $(B♀ \times A♂)F_1$ hybrids. Although both of these classes of "reciprocal" hybrids have exactly similar genetic constitutions, they differ with regard to the maternal environment in which they were gestated (see Fig. 15-2).

Adult individuals belonging to both classes of hybrids and produced by mating homozygous parents from two different strains were lethally irradiated and rehabilitated by infusion of bone marrow "grafts" from a donor of one or other of the two parental strains, and the delayed mortality due to graft-versus-host reactivity was then evaluated. It was found that the severity of these reactions was significantly reduced if the marrow donor was syngeneic with the female parent that gestated the F_1 hybrid, indicating a reduction in the antigenicity in the host. For example, when RIII strain bone marrow cells were injected into lethally irradiated (C57BL $\times$ RIII)F_1 hybrid recipients, the cumulative mortality was 50%; but with the reciprocal (RIII $\times$ C57BL)F_1 hybrid recipients of RIII marrow the cumulative mortality was only 20%.

RECIPROCAL HYBRID EXPERIMENT

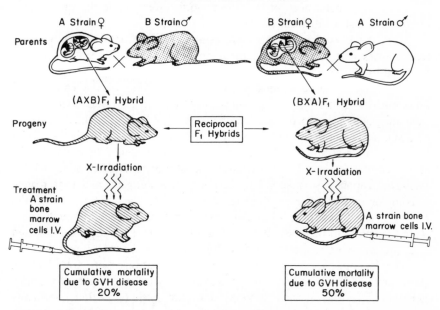

Fig. 15-2. Illustrating the production of reciprocal hybrid mice who are genetically identical but differ with regard to the maternal genetic milieu in which they are gestated. This figure illustrates the differential susceptibility of the two classes of F_1 hybrids to graft-versus-host disease following irradiation and inoculation with bone marrow cells from one of the parental strains.

Not all parental strains, or rather their marrow cells, were able to "recognize" this subtle quantitative reduction of antigenicity in the F_1 hybrid host. It was found, however, that parental strains that were unable to recognize these maternally acquired differences in antigenicity of reciprocal hybrids could be made to do so by interposing an additional experimental procedure before marrow transplantation. This entailed exposure of the parental strain donor bone marrow cells to washed erythrocytes from one or other of the reciprocal F_1 hybrids, before injection into the lethally irradiated subjects. This resulted in an increased or decreased incidence of fatal graft-versus-host disease depending on whether the antigenicity of the "priming" stimulus to which the donor marrow cells was exposed *in vitro* was greater or less than the host's antigenicity. Marrow from both parental strains caused more severe graft-versus-host reactivity following *in vitro* sensitization when the erythrocytes were obtained from a hybrid donor whose mother was allogeneic to the donor of the marrow cells. This indicated that these cells were qualitatively more antigenic than genetically similar cells from the reciprocal hybrid.

2. *Ova-transfer substrains* were established by transferring homozygous fertilized eggs from a female of one genotype to the uterus of an appropriate female of a different genotype. Subsequently, an "adapted" male and an "adapted" female born of the foster mother were made the progenitors of an ova-transfer substrain (see Fig. 15-3).

3. *Foster-nursed substrains* were established by Caesarean delivery of term fetuses and foster nursing them on homozygous allogeneic females, followed by inbreeding as above.

Experimental studies, mostly entailing evaluation of the capacity of bone marrow grafts from these substrains to elicit graft-versus-host reactions in genetically appropriate irradiated test hosts, have yielded evidence of a significantly diminished capacity to respond to tissue antigens of the foster mother's strain. Dr. Uphoff also obtained evidence that, with some strain combinations, the ova-transfer substrain individual acquired an *increased* capacity to respond to certain tissue antigens and that foster-nursing or ova transfer resulted in alterations in the antigenicity of the hosts' tissues from those of the original ancestral strain. Although these were too subtle to be detected by skin grafting tests, they could be detected with the aid of bone marrow grafts along the lines described above.

The fact that these various phenotypic alterations were found to be permanent and vertically transmitted from mother to progeny for many generations in the derived sublines does not entirely exclude vertically transmitted alien cells from the original foster mother as a contributory factor, though it seems unlikely.

On the basis of these interesting findings Uphoff has proposed that the basic mechanism responsible for these maternally induced alterations in

PRODUCTION OF OVA TRANSFER SUBSTRAIN

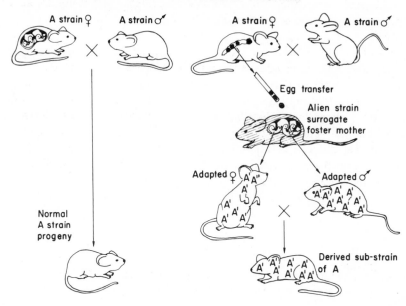

Fig. 15-3. Showing the production of an ova-transfer substrain by transferring homozygous fertilized eggs from a female of one genotype to the endocrinologically prepared uterus of a female of an unrelated genotype. Subsequently an adapted "foster gestated and nursed" brother and sister are mated to produce the derived substrain. Animals of the adapted substrain differ from the strain from which they originated by subtle differences in the phenotypic expression of both the immunogenicity of their tissues and their immunologic responses to allografts.

antigenicity of the tissues of the progeny and the altered responsiveness of these individuals toward tissue antigens have evolved through selective advantages associated with preventing rejection of the fetus as an allograft.

Conclusions

The influence of antigenic disparities with respect to the various series of alloantigens, between the conceptus and the mother, as well as the immunologic status of the latter with regard to them on overall fertility, sex ratio, and the maintenance of the polymorphisms concerned is a subject urgently in need of carefully designed investigations rather than facile armchair speculation. Particularly important in this regard is the fact that man appears to have a Y-linked histocompatibility antigen that is expressed by spermatozoa and possibly by early zygotes as well. No evidence exists that maternal HL-A antibodies in general have any untoward effects on the fetus and there are no convincing indications of an association of a high proportion of stillbirths or abortions with maternal HL-A sensitization. A comprehensive search has yet to be made for evidence of fertility differences connected with different levels of HL-A incompatibility between conceptuses and their mothers.

On a slight facetious note, at a time in history when overproduction of mankind appears to be endangering the species, pregnancy may be regarded as a venereal disease. The balance of currently available evidence seems to hint that polymorphism with regard to at least some systems of cell surface alloantigens contributes to the incidence of this disease so far as its "clinical" manifestation is concerned. It is ironical that with many conventional diseases of microbial origin various authors have presented cogent arguments that host cell membrane antigenic polymorphisms play or have played an important role in resistance.

R E F E R E N C E S

"Biological significance of histocompatibility antigens." 1972. Fogerty International Center Proceedings, No. 15. *Fed. Proc.* **31**:1087–1104.

Clarke, B., and Kirby, D. R. S. 1966. "Maintenance of histocompatibility polymorphisms." *Nature* (London) **211**:999–1000.

Cloudman, A. M. 1941. "The effect of an extra-chromosomal influence upon transplanted spontaneous tumors in mice." *Science* **93**:380–381.

Green, I. 1974. "Genetic control of immune responses." *Immunogenetics* **1**:4–21.

Hull, P. 1969. "Maternal-fetal incompatibility associated with the H-3 locus in the mouse." *Heredity* **24**:203–209.

Jackson, C. E., Mann, J. D., and Shull, W. J. 1969. "Xg^a blood group system and the sex ratio in man." *Nature* (London) **222**:445–446.

Kirby, D. R. S. 1970. "The egg and immunology." *Proc. Roy. Soc. Med.* **63**: 59–61.

Kirby, D. R. S., McWhirter, K. G., Teitelbaum, M. S., and Darlington, C. D. 1967. "A possible immunological influence on sex ratio." *Lancet* **ii**: 139–140.

Lappé, M., and Schalk, J. 1971. "Necessity of the spleen for balanced secondary sex ratios following maternal immunization with male antigen." *Transplantation* **11**:491–495.

Law, L. W. 1942. "Foster nursing and the growth of transplantable leukemias in mice." *Can. Res.* **2**:108–115.

McLaren, A. 1962. "Does immunity to male antigen affect female reproductive performance?" *Nature* (London) **195**:1323–1324.

Matsunaga, E., and Itoh, S. 1957. "Blood groups and fertility in a Japanese population, with special reference to intra-uterine selection due to maternal-foetal incompatibility." *Ann. Human Genet.* **22**:111–131.

Palm, J. 1970. "Maternal-fetal interactions and histocompatibility antigen polymorphisms." *Transpl. Proc.* **2**:162–173.

Palm, J. 1974. "Maternal-fetal histoincompatibility in rats—an escape from adversity." *Can. Res.* **34**:2061–2065.

Renkonen, K. O., Mäkelä, O., and Lehtovaara, R. 1962. "Factors affecting the human sex ratio." *Nature* (London) **194**:308–309.

Scott, J. R., and Beer, A. E. 1973. "Immunological factors in first pregnancy Rh immunisation." *Lancet* **i**:717–718.

Stern, C. 1973. *Principles of human genetics,* 3rd ed. W. H. Freeman, San Francisco, Calif.

Toivanen, P., and Hirvonen, T. 1970. "Sex ratio of newborns: Preponderance of male in toxemia of pregnancy." *Science* **170**:187–188.

Uphoff, D. E. 1973. "Maternal influences on mouse embryos and preservation of mutant mouse strains by freezing." *Science* **181**:287–288.

Uphoff, D. E. 1973. "Maternal influences on the immune response." *Biomedicine* **18**:13–22.

Wachtel, S. S., Koo, G. C., Zuckerman, E. E., Hammerling, U., Scheid, M. P., and Boyse, E. A. 1974. "Serologic crossreactivity between H-Y (male) antigens of mouse and man." *Proc. Nat. Acad. Sci.* **71**:1215–1218.

Index

ABO antibodies:
  presence in milk, 201–204
  role in hemolytic disease, 157
  role in infertility, 71
ABO antigens:
  in hemolytic disease of newborn, 150, 156
  in incompatible marriages, 222, 225
  ontogeny of, 226
Abortion:
  ALS-induced, 111
  resulting from maternal sensitization, 160, 171, 223, 231
  spontaneous, 223
Abortuses, sex of, 224
Adoptive immunization, through suckling, 211, 213
Allograft reaction, 14
Allophenic mice, 141, 143
Allotypes, 49
  suppression of, 159
Amniotic fluid, 195
Anterior chamber, as graft site, 11
Antibodies (*see also* ABO antibodies and Rh):
  appearance in newborn, 177
  "blocking" (*see also* Immunoregulation), 47, 116, 126, 131, 142, 156, 169, 227
  copro-antibodies, 203
  cytotoxic, 46
  effect on sex ratio, 227
  HL-A in multiparous women, 156
  IgA, in colostrum and milk, 6
  IgE, 192, 195
  IgG, 181, 192, 193, 195
  IgM, 181, 192, 193, 195
  to leukocytes—influence on fetal development, 158
  to platelets, 158
  against spermatozoa, 52, 56, 62, 66, 67
  in uterine fluid, 192
Antigens:
  accessory male reproductive glands, 60
  blood group (*see* ABO antigens and Rh)
  brain, 45, 52, 60, 68, 108
  cardiac muscle, 44
  casein, 44
  kidney, 109, 116
  lens, 43, 108

Antigens (*cont.*)
  milk, 44
  placenta, 116
  role in maturation of lymphoid tissue, 179
  semen, 52
  sequestered, 43, 52
  spermatozoal, 52, 67, 69, 70, 71, 82
  testicular, 44, 54, 55, 59, 108, 116
  thyroglobulin, 43
  transplantation, ontogeny of, 87, 182
Antilymphocyte serum (ALS), 48
Antiplacental serum, 108 *et seq.*
Armadillos:
  choriocarcinoma in, 105
  quadruplets in, 143
Aspermatogenesis:
  of immunologic etiology, 56
  prevention of, 59
  role of antibodies, 63
Autoimmune diseases, 41
  encephalomyelitis, 45, 59, 60
  glomerulonephritis, 45
  Hashimoto's, 41, 45
  influence of pregnancy on, 120
  role of suppressor T cells in, 49
  role of T and B lymphocytes in, 44
  systemic lupus erythematosis, 49
  transmissibility of, 44, 45
Autoimmunity:
  against adrenal gland, 45
  influence of blocking antibodies on, 47, 118
  against semen, 69
  against testis, 1, 45, 56, 60
  thyroid, 41, 45

Barrier:
  blood-mammary gland, 201
  blood-testis, 56, 57, 74
  placental, 85
Blastocyst, 10, 11, 110
  antigens of, 82
  development of, 12
  fluid, 13, 15
  interspecific transfer, 89, 90
  intraspecific transfer, 11, 77, 88, 114, 141, 218
  zona-free, 94
Blastokinin, 10

235